Natural Home Remedies That Will Help You with Everyday Illnesses

By Michael Persaud

This book is dedicated to my wife, parents, and siblings, who have always supported me in whatever I choose to do. Special love goes to our cat, Ashleigh, who fills my heart with a lot of love from just looking at his cute face. It is also dedicated to those people who like to make a concerted effort of taking care of their health and being proactive rather than reactive.

Table of Contents

Preface

I decided to write this book in order to help people with everyday ailments which they are sometimes not mentally equipped to deal with. Yes, doctors have a lot of experience dealing with sick people, but they might not always have the solution to remedy various ailments. And for everyone one size does not fit all. I know from having a half a century of dealing with doctors for various ailments. Unfortunately, sometimes they are way off in their prognosis.

During my half century on this planet I've come across a lot of people either in school (high school or college), the working world, through friends and associates, family, and people who I've met through family members. Some of them disclose ailments they suffer from and how they best cope with their symptoms. Some have gone to doctors but still cannot find a solution to their problems. True, doctors have many years of schooling and training, but they don't always know the answers.

I have spoken to many people and found out what they do in order to help themselves when medical science is unable to do so. I will suggest natural things that you can purchase at your grocery or drug stores that do not require a prescription. **Full disclose: I'm not getting paid by the company of any product which I am endorsing, I just believe they work when sometimes medical science fails us.** Not everyone's body is the same although humans share a common DNA, and sometimes when one medication will work for others, it will have minimal or no effect on other people. I know from experience and from what other people disclose to me. If you've lived with an ailment you will know it more intimately than your family physician. God bless them; however, doctors may sometimes steer you wrong. I've had it happen numerous times. The best advice I've actually gotten were from lay people, who have actually had the ailment from which I may be suffering from, at that particular time.

In this book I will mention products or natural remedies for such things as constipation, alopecia (hair loss), hearing loss, upset stomachs, urinary infections, diarrhea and others when prescription medications fail to help. I hope to help you too as I've found them to be very helpful in my existence and others I've associated in this world. I should add that some of these remedies have been divulged by doctors as well, when they do not provide a prescription for some medication, at the time you are suffering from any specific ailment.

Full disclosure: I have been prescribed some medications that made me even sicker or given medications which had nothing to do with my ailment. That could have proven to be disastrous or even fatal had I taken the medication. Keep in mind, doctors and pharmacists are only human, and there are limitations to their knowledge and expertise. A few times I have had to visit several doctors before I received a proper diagnosis. Doctors take an educated guess when you visit them. They are not clairvoyants. But I should mention there are a lot of great doctors out there. My current family physician is amazing, I might add.

Thank you for purchasing this book, I hope it comes in very useful when you are trying to help yourself to find some relief, or a cure, and modern medical practices are not helping.

Also I've learned some of these suggestions by reading medical articles for 32 years, usually about twice a week so in 32 years that would 32 years x 2 articles x 52 weeks = 3,328 articles which originate from such medical journals as The Lancet (the British medical journal), JAMA (Journal of the American Medical Association), and doctors who are interviewed in the newspaper or who either write their own opinion columns. That being said, on the nightly news there are usually medical stories which have some great advice where doctors are being interviewed where I have gleaned some excellent tips. That's over the same 32-year period (that's again about 3,328 TV medical reports, not to mention TV news programs where doctors are interviewed concerning their area of expertise). No, I'm not against the medical world they are a great boon to society as a whole, but sometimes there are times when it fails us. *That being said, if you are suffering from some really serious ailment like cancer, multiple sclerosis, Parkinson's, influenza,*

Alzheimer's, or maybe pneumonia or bronchitis, please seek medical help. What I disclose here may augment your treatment.

Also, as we age 40-years-old is usually the age when our bodies peak and start to change, that is when most of us start going grey, need to wear glasses, begin to lose muscle mass, and our memory starts to fade.

I hope this book comes in useful for you. I thank all the people who have imparted their experience about their ailments over the past 32 plus years. They have lived their illnesses and not learned about it second hand. Sometimes experience is the best teacher of all.

Chapter 1

Urinary Tract Infections

Urinary tract infections are one thing that will affect either men or women at some time in their lives. You can tell when you have one as you will feel your urethra having a very uncomfortable feeling. It might feel that something is impeding the way when you are about to urinate or you might experience just total discomfort.

I use to suffer from it in my early forties. Something that works like a charm is pure cranberry juice like from Ocean Spray. Remember this is not cranberry drink which is impure. It's ***pure cranberry juice*** which you need to alleviate the problem.

My wife has had urinary tract infections as well and **Ocean Spray cranberry juice** works almost like magic. Just have a glass and you will see that when you urinate it will coat the inside of your urinary tract and your problem will be gone within day.

When I've had had urinary tract infections, I always headed for the Ocean Spray. There are some medications which your pharmacist can give you, one I believe is a pill form, but that will not do the trick as it is *not pure cranberry juice.* Natural things work better sometimes rather than the synthetic form.

Pure cranberry juice works extremely well. My wife and I swear by it. Once in my life I kept getting urinary tract infections every several months and, yes, it may have been because I was sexually active – after all I am married – and every single time Ocean Spray cranberry juice worked like magic. I would swear by it. That being said, if your urinary problem persists over 2-days I would highly recommend seeing a doctor to see if your health issue is not more serious. (Especially if you see blood in your urine.) But my urinary problems have sometimes gone away within less than a day after drinking pure cranberry juice. Sometimes the Almighty puts natural things within our grasp to help us mortal humans with issues we might have.

Chapter 2

Upset Stomachs

We, as humans, like to consume a lot of different kinds of foods. Since all of our bodies are not the same, some foods may affect some people, but not others. That's why celiacs who are allergic to gluten can get really sick if they consume wheat-based products. That's not to fault them, their biology is just different than other humans.

I've known people in my life who have consumed bread with gluten all their lives. One of my colleagues developed gluten intolerance when he hit his forties. Another friend at the age of fifty was diagnosed with gluten intolerance. Both of these people had consumed bread with gluten their entire lives and did not have a problem. They both just developed gluten intolerance as they aged.

A person who is a celiac and who cannot tolerate gluten-based products can get stomach cramps and even diarrhea if they are not careful what they eat. Since gluten intolerance is a growing problem a lot of restaurants will have special entrees for people with this allergy. My one colleague will not eat out in restaurants any longer as there have been mix-ups with his foods at some restaurants and he has gotten terribly ill. He'd rather make his own meals at home and is now an avid cook.

Now getting back to the focus of this chapter. Since we consume various foods, some of which may not agree with us, or sometimes have food poisoning from undercooked foods, or in some cases I've had some friends who love barbecue meats but can't tolerate the BBQ sauce, there is a remedy for someone who has an upset stomach. **That magic elixir is Canada Dry Ginger Ale**. That product is one of the magic items sitting on our grocery shelves. Sprite or Mountain Dew will not do the trick. If you have an upset stomach and may even have diarrhea, open a can or bottle of Canada Dry Ginger Ale and let the fizz of bubbles dissipate. That's called making the drink "flat". When that happens the Canada Dry Ginger Ale is more potent for helping someone with an upset stomach. It takes some time to work but can work within a day. I'm surprised some pharmacies don't sell this product because it works better than a prescription drug and, of course, would be less toxic to your system. The excess which you consume which does not end up in your stomach or bladder you will just urinate out. And it costs less than a prescription drug and you can you buy it at any corner store.

Mountain Dew like Sprite will not cure an upset stomach. If someone tells you so – don't believe them! Those two drinks will not work. Sure, both of these two drinks are great to consume on social occasions, but it's the ginger in Canada Dry Ginger Ale that coats your stomach and adding to the healing of your stomach.

However, if you are gluten intolerant or lactose intolerant (allergic to diary products), you might still need Canada Dry Ginger Ale if you happen to get diarrhea. When your stomach starts to heal if you have eaten dairy, unmistakably, or there is some gluten in your meal which has been included accidentally, Canada Dry Ginger Ale will still help. There are some people who can tolerate some dairy products but not others. I can tolerate most any dairy product but there are some which affect me. I can consume most yogurts and ice cream and milk products, but there are some dairy products which will cause me to have diarrhea, and send me running for the nearest lavatory.

Also, if you have uncontrollable runs and if the product Imodium is not helping, you might have to go on the **BRAT Diet**. This one is sanctioned by the medical community. Below is what the acronym BRAT stands for:

B – Bananas

R – Rice, plain white rice

A – Applesauce

T – Toast, or bread (white bread, not whole wheat, as the latter has fiber which will produce bowel movements)

Most of what is in the BRAT diet will bind your stool and will stop you from going to the washroom frequently. Having said that, applesauce does not always work for everyone. I once was on the BRAT diet and when I consumed applesauce it literally went right through me. So, applesauce may not work for you either. But, if it does, more power to you!

Children who have upset stomachs usually are put on the BRAT Diet by doctors. A former business associate of mine and I bonded once discussing the BRAT Diet as her young daughter had to go on it several times.

As you see everything in the BRAT Diet can be purchased from your local grocery store without a prescription and most of it is all natural. Most of it will cost less than a prescription. Of course, the applesauce can sometimes be processed. The others are right from nature. However, again if your stomach ailments persist please see a doctor to ensure that your stomach issues are not more serious. I have to say though that going on the BRAT diet has always worked like a charm for me.

Just yesterday I had a terrible upset stomach from consuming bad plums the night before. Our extended family was headed to a great Italian restaurant to celebrate my wife's and my wedding anniversary. A few hours before I had a can of Canady Dry Ginger Ale, which my wife rushed out to buy me at the corner store, and by the time supper rolled around, my stomach was almost back to normal, and I was able to enjoy a delicious entrée of chicken cacciatore.

One last thing is eating white rice might not be the most tasteful thing, so if you want to mix in a little sardine to add some flavor it might make the taste more palatable.

Chapter 3

Hair Loss

As we age hair loss is one thing men and women will suffer from. The technical term used to refer to hair loss in both men and women is alopecia. Some people may even see it in their late adolescence (usually males) or while they enter their early twenties.

It is said that we usually inherit our hair lines from our mothers, meaning that if your mother has lush thick hair, her children too will inherit good and beautiful lush hair. I have generally found that to be an Old Wives' Tale, as there are some young men who have bald men on their mother's side of the family, but they still have a great head of hair well into middle-age and beyond. Conversely, the opposite I have found to be true as well. Some guys I have known have great hairlines on their mother's side of the family but prematurely lost their hair into their twenties.

There is also another factor which I've observed from empirical observation in my life. It was surprising that an aunt of mine who lives in the United States, also has the same conjecture, as she noticed the same phenomenon as she aged. She's in her mid-sixties now and retired.

What is that phenomenon?: it was men who used gel or hair products but mostly gel. Since my adolescence I've noticed my contemporaries in my teens who used gel, but as they continued to use it for many years, they started to lose hair follicles. Their fathers however were not bald nor did their mothers possess alopecia or thinning hair.

They were men of various ethnicities who used gel, in my milieu, while growing up, and the more they used it, the more their hair thinned. Herewith, I will mention the men who lost their hair, and some of whom had very thick hair, but as they continued to used copious amounts of gel, they lost more and more hair.

Here are their names and ethnicities, Stephen (half Spanish and half Hungarian), Faud (half Indian and half Afghani), Tom (Greek), Yogi (Indian), Peter (Irish and German), Kai (half Indian and half Caucasian), and Joseph (Indian). The aforesaid males all had thick hair but continued to use gel from their teens well into their twenties and early thirties. There was a black gentleman who I knew in his twenties who shaved his head, I am not sure if he lost his hair, or was just doing it as a fashion statement. He's in his forties right now and still shaves his head, ergo, I conjecture he might have been going bald. I don't know if he ever used gel or hair products. But he is a contemporary of mine so there is a possibility he might have. Simon (Irish) and Dave (British) also lost their hair but Simon and Dave always had thinning hair and did not use gel. The others all used copious amounts of gel for many years. Some had really lush and thick hair but it all started to fall out while they were in their twenties or just as they reached 30-years-of-age. Most of their fathers had great heads of hair into their twilight years.

My aunt Cecilia noticed this phenomenon for many years while residing in the United States (and still does), she disclosed to me that all the men she knew who used gel for many years after several years all became bald. Her and I never spoke about this for decades, but my conjecture was solidified after we had a conversation over the phone one day when I reached middle-age. I had noticed this strange phenomenon during the course of 30 years as did she.

After her and conversed, I was certain that my conjecture was correct.

Now, how do you remedy or lessen the loss of hair? Keep in mind, there are some middle-aged women or those in their twilight years who have thinning hair. I have an older female relative who was also experiencing hair loss until someone told her about a vitamin, that she can purchase over the counter at her drug store, which restored much of her hair. What is that product? **It's Vitamin B12**. That same relative disclosed it to me as she noticed that I started to have thinning hair. And truth be known after I started to take Vitamin B12 my thinning hair is beginning to look lusher after a few weeks. My female relative's hair started to thin 10 years ago. She's in her seventies now and her hair has been restored. And all she did was start taking Vitamin B12.

I spoke with my pharmacist, and he said that Vitamin B12 is safe to take, because what our body does not use, the remainder will be passed out of our bodies when we urinate.

I take 1000 mcg (micro grams) each day and have been for several weeks now. It's been working like a charm.

My female elderly relative's hair has also been restored mostly but is thicker than when she started to lose it. I'm sorry I can't give credit where credit is due as my relative does not recall who told her to take B12. My elderly relative is about 74 years of age now, so it is never too late to start taking B12. One word of caution: take B12 in the morning as it may also give you a boost of energy so if you take it closer to bed you may not able to fall asleep. I have to admit I initially had this problem when I first started taking it – although I took it in the morning with breakfast – but since my body got acclimated to it, I fall asleep at night now like a baby.

So, if you're suffering from alopecia, I recommend using Vitamin B12, it's harmless and what your body does not use will be passed out of your system when you urinate. What have you got to lose? It's harmless, can be purchased over the counter at your local pharmacy, and you will not have to get a hair transplant or wear a wig. It's a win-win situation!

Chapter 4
Stress Relievers

North Americans and those in the Western World work long hours. That being said, South Koreans and the Japanese work really long hours as well. In Japan there is a term for death by overwork, it is called karoshi. There are no reported incidents of karoshi in North American but it is quite prevalent in Japan. They also have a name for "constant improvement" which is kaizen. The more you become adept at something, the better you are able to perform that task with little effort, and become better organized at doing it. But sometimes kaizen can lead to karoshi if a person is spending long hours at the office working, with little sleep or little leisure time, to recharge their internal batteries.

In America some companies do not guarantee a worker a set vacation time each year. If a worker needs to take time off, they might have to lose pay. In Canada once a worker starts a job, they are guaranteed at least 2 weeks vacation time each year. Also, in America there is no guarantee maternity leave for new mothers. In Canada, a new mother now gets a year and a half off with reduced pay. That time can be shared between the mother and father of a new born.

In Europe it is somewhat of a very different scenario. New workers at a company are guaranteed at sometimes 5 or 6 weeks vacation each year. I use to have 5 weeks at one of my last companies due to my being there for 20 years. It was a luxury, and I have to admit, I did log into my work computer to do work, even when on vacation, as I could not find things to do if I was not going out of town for a trip. That was a sweet deal. Unfortunately, most workers do not see that much vacation time in one year.

There should be a work-life balance for all workers. Most of our days are very stressful with deadlines to meet, meetings to attend, fighting commuter traffic every day, meeting quotas, seminars to attend, or travelling for conferences outside of our city or state or province or country. That can take a toll especially if you will be travelling through different time zones which can lead to jet lag. Take it from me – as I've had to do this before – if travelling through different time zones for your job, sign up for a personal day or a vacation day (if you can), or work from home when you return back to your house, apartment, or condo, as your body will be enervated, and it will take some time for you to get acclimated back to your regular time zone and your biological clock. I travelled with a colleague once to a conference through 4 time zones, and she shrewdly suggested I take a day off, when I returned back to our home city. Her advice was truly a blessing.

Getting back to the stress factor at work. Everyone needs a work-life balance from their hectic days. It seems more people are becoming stressed during their daily jobs. Sometimes working overtime or doing additional weekend work can take a toll on the body and mind. Everyone needs some downtime to recharge and re-energize. Weekends are good for that.

Some things to do to help you alleviate stress is to go for a jog or a walk after work. If there is inclement weather like thunderstorms, or tremendous snow and ice, you can always join a gym and use their treadmills. Or if you live in a condo you can use the gym in your building, or you may wish to invest in one for your home. You can also kill two birds with one stone by watching TV when you walk, listen to music, or some people choose to listen to audio books for entertainment purposes, or to learn something new that may benefit them personally or with their jobs. It's great to pass the time and you will not notice the time going by. If you don't keep your mind occupied while working out, the workout can maybe feel like drudgery or a real chore, and may actually be de-motivating. That would be counterproductive to de-stressing from a hard day at the office.

You could also do laundry or read the newspaper or read a book or watch a sitcom or movie on your iPad.

Journaling can be a good stress reliever too. It's very cathartic because you will be relieving mental tension. I've tried this before and it works extremely well. Once

I was very upset at cyclists on the sidewalk who make it perilous for pedestrians. I was very angry and went home and wrote about it. After I was done ranting on paper, I felt 100% better. I was surprised at how much it changed my mindset. Journaling is also like speaking to a person or a psychologist or psychiatrist without getting any feedback.

You could also go for a bike ride or use a stationary bicycle. The tension it relieves is remarkable. Be sure to wear a helmet, elbow and knee pads for your protection. When I was in my twenties and thirties, I use to use a stationary bike at home every day after work. It was great exercise and an excellent stress reliever.

You could choose to write a book, read one, or try your hand at some art. You could sketch or paint abstracts, still life, or copy from the newspaper. We all learn by copying other people. That's how we first started to learn to speak, walk, or behave when we were young – by watching and learning from our parents or siblings, cousins, or aunts and uncles.

There are some people who enjoy crafts. That might be a good option for you as well.

Or call up a friend or relative. If your friend or relative has a great sense of humor you might be in for a laugh session. I've had a couple of friends in the past who have had great rapier wits who always had me in stitches. They were great to banter with.

Or watch a movie on Netflix. If you can't afford Netflix borrow a DVD from your local library or a friend.

If you choose to go on social media like Facebook, that might relieve some tension, but keep in mind you might see some of your Facebook friends who are having fabulous lives which may have a negative effect on your mental outlook. Keep in mind, most people curate their Facebook pages to make it appear that they are having the best life ever. Not true, everyone has trials and tribulations as some of my Facebook friends have disclosed to me. Twitter, is great at expressing yourself but I've found lately that there are some people on Twitter who are very negative and who only write abusive things to others. I can count on one hand 3 of my Facebook friends who mostly put negative comments on things I post. I know most of them are self-aggrandizing, and I've seen it come back to bite them, so seeing that Karma in action is a pleasure in and of itself.

Or you could join a book club. You might enjoy the intricacies or plots of a novel. Plus, every time you meet it will be a social event, where you can meet new and refreshing people, if your coworkers are the ones who are causing you stress.

If you're the active kind, why not join a basketball, hockey, baseball, flag football, frisbee football, poker group, investing group (yes, you will have the potential to make more money!), or take some classes at your local community college or university.

Museums offer free lectures on many interesting topics, by some very engaging experts, where you can learn about something new which will broaden your mind. Some museums may also offer some classes where you are actively engaged like with pottery, painting, or sketching.

There are many things you can do outside of work which can offer relief from stress. You might also want to change vocations so you could take some night school courses which can lead to a diploma or certificate.

Ever want to learn a new language or learn to play a musical instrument? There are classes offered at night either privately or at your local high school or college or university.

Why not start a film club where you and other film buffs can keep up on the latest movies coming out of Hollywood or foreign films?

The world is your oyster. I'm sure you can think of many other options which can interest you and which can lead to stress relief. These are just some choices to get you started.

Chapter 5
Taking Care of Your Bowels

Everyone should take care of their bowels as they must have it for life. There is a problem in our society where we eat a lot of rich foods which are great tasting but which are not beneficial to our bowels. There are proctology clinics which are filled with people of all races and ages who have issues with their bowels. Not all of them have the same problems with their bowels.

Most of bowel problems stem from what we consume. There was a young lady I knew who drank a lot of Coke which is not good for you. There are 5 table spoons of sugar in each can of Coke. Every time she would consume a can of Coke or Pepsi, she would have diarrhea the next morning. Still she refused to acknowledge that the soda was causing her problem.

We, as a society, do not eat a lot of whole grains, or nuts, or fruits and vegetables. If you think you can't afford it there are cheap grocery stores which sell fruits and vegetables at affordable prices. If you live in a large city and you have a Chinatown, you can get those items there for a steal. So, there is no excuse for not consuming fruits, vegetables, or nuts which produce good bacteria in your bowels. And in order to have a healthy bowel and good bowel movements you need to eat healthy things. They are also a great source of fiber which we need as human beings. Our ancestors consumed a lot of those before the Industrial Revolution, because when their economies and livelihoods were more agrarian (dealing with agriculture), they lived off the land and ate more fruits and vegetables.

Most people today eat a lot of fast foods and processed foods. Most of the foods on our grocery shelves in boxes or cans are processed which is not good for us. Sure, they may be good to eat for their taste and flavor, but you have to remember eat everything in moderation.

A lot of people due to their busy lives eat a lot of take-out like pizza, Chinese food, Indian food, burgers, fries, and chicken wings from fast food outlets. Sure, they taste great but eating those kinds of foods every night will not bode well for good bowel health. If you consume those food products do so in moderation, but you should also consume fruits, vegetables, and nuts every night. A handful of raw almonds is good for your cholesterol level but it will also contribute to good bowel movements.

Some people who have an enormous problem with too much diarrhea, or bad bacteria in their bowels, actually have had feces implanted in their bowels which can sometimes rectify their problem. What this means is that doctors will collect feces from a person with good bacteria in their bowels, and actually place it inside the bowels of someone with bowel problems (who most likely has bad bacteria in their bowel). It's a new and innovative procedure but it does work for some people.

Also eat yogurt with probiotics. That will contribute to having good bacteria in your bowels. And if you're not lactose intolerant it might help you if you have bowel issues.

My wife and I add a crudité or salad to our meals every night. A crudité is basically cut up vegetables which we consume by dipping into hummus. You can cut up all sorts of vegetables like carrots, celery, radishes, green, red, or orange bell peppers, cherry tomatoes, or cucumbers. It all tastes great! At first, I was not too big on radishes but I have grown to really love them.

Or you can have salad with some very nice salad dressing. That is good fiber and as they say good "roughage" will produce excellent bowel movements.

I have found the older I get I can tolerate processed foods even less. Sure, I do indulge in Chinese, Greek, Jamaican, Indian, pizza, wings, and other foods which are not suppose to be too good for you. Yes, Chinese food has a lot of MSG (monosodium glutamate), but it does taste great! I consume the aforesaid foods in moderation and I usually have good bowel movements. One of the best feelings in the world is to have a good bowel movement, because on the other end of the spectrum, having constipation is not pleasant at all.

Constipation can leave a person feeling bloated, internally obstructed, and having much discomfort.

With beverages, again moderation is the key. You can consume beer, wine, alcohol, and sodas, but please do it again in moderation. Whenever we consume something to an excess it leads to an imbalance within us. And that is not good for a good function digestive system. I have witnessed some families at the grocery store purchasing cases of soda sometimes. I think to myself but are they doing any good to their health? (Some of those families are carrying an excess of weight – both the parents and children. Children today already get a very inadequate amount of exercise due to them having a lot of screen time on their phones, tablets, computer, and sitting for hours in front of the TV.) You can consume those beverages every once in a while, but not every day. I once worked with a gentleman who was overweight. He always drank a can of soda every day with his lunch. I think that added to his being overweight and in the long run will be detrimental to his health leading to conditions like diabetes. He was already in his sixties.

If you're going to have some wine with dinner, indulge in it a little, don't polish off a bottle every night. Also, all those beverages have a lot of sugar which is not good when it sits on your teeth for too long. Coffee and tea will give you a mental boost, and more clarity of mind during the working day, but be sure to rinse your mouth after consuming them as they will stain your teeth.

Flavonoids are what gives fruits and vegetables their color and pigment. The richer the flavonoids on a fruit or vegetable, the better they are for you because flavonoids are a great antioxidant as well.

But please remember to add more fruits, vegetables, and nuts (walnuts, raw almonds, peanuts, sunflower seeds) to your diet. When it comes to grapes and watermelons eat those in moderation as well as they contain a lot of sugar which can lead to diabetes. Same with orange or apple juice. They have a lot of sugar. Moderation is the key. But remember to drink milk every day as you have to maintain strong bones. Spinach is also a good source of calcium just like milk.

It's better to get vitamins naturally from nature than in the synthetic pill form.

Red meat is not that good for you like beef, lamb, pork, and duck. Yes, I was surprised to find that duck meat is red meat as well. Too much red meat can lead to bowel problems and maybe even cancer of the rectum or colon. Colorectal cancer is one of the leading killers of North Americans today. And people of all ages can get it.

Chicken, turkey, and fish are good for you. Lean chicken meat, fish like salmon, tuna, or sardines are great for you. But with the canned fish moderation again is the key as they may contain too much mercury. Too much mercury in our system can be detrimental to maintaining good health.

A person with a healthy bowel is a person who is happy. And that's what you're aiming for.

(I would like to address the issue of being overweight again. With obesity usually comes things like high blood pressure, too much bad cholesterol, and diabetes due to inactivity. However, there are a small minority of obese people who do not suffer from any of those conditions. Those people are healthy and doctors call the condition the "obesity paradox." I should mention that those who have the obesity paradox are in the minority. Thin people can look healthy but can still suffer from high blood pressure, too much bad cholesterol, and diabetes.)

Chapter 6
Migraines

Migraines can be very problematic for many people. I had a school chum named Simon who had them from a very early age, in fact, since we were in middle school (then called junior high). He also had it throughout high school but, alas, we lost touch after high school. I know when he had it, he was in excruciating mental anguish, and was often driven to tears due to the mental pain he felt. He had seen doctors but there was no relief.

In my adult life I've had some colleagues who suffered from migraines, and still they could not find a remedy for a condition, which has been around for many decades. Yes, doctors can prescribe Tylenol or Advil but it might be a temporary relief until the pain subsides.

What triggers it? Being in fluorescent light could be one trigger; the barometer changing when it is about to rain could be another; stress from work can cause it as well; even studying for a lot of exams could lead to it; even consuming alcohol for some people could trigger them; or sometimes migraines can surface without warning. For those who suffer from it, it is no a laughing matter. The pain they feel can send them to their beds for the evening or even for a number of days depending on the mental anguish they feel.

I have a friend who also suffers from it. It runs in the family as both her mother and her suffer from years of having migraines, so it is in her DNA and she inherited the condition from her beloved mother. Her mother would sometimes take several Tylenol to relieve the mental pain, which would subside after a few hours or a few days, but would lead to another problem: constipation. The Tylenol would lead to her being incapable of having bowel movements which was the results of her taking too many Tylenols.

My friend Sarah, has had migraines since she was a child. She is a very intelligent young lady who speaks two languages and has great self-taught culinary talents. She's also very sociable and has a good circle of friends. She enjoys reading, the movies, the theatre, concerts, cooking, and baking and one of her past times is travelling the world.

That makes for a full life. But Sarah has been beset all her life with the nagging problem of migraines. When they come on, they come on very strong. The things which usually triggered hers in the present and the past were: lack of sleep; having a stressful day at work; being in too much fluorescent light; processed foods; being dehydrated especially when she sometimes consumes too much alcohol; spending too much time on her phone or in front of the computer and exposing her brain to too much light; hormonal changes within her body; overusing medication; drinking too much caffeine (yes, we're a caffeine culture who spend a lot of time in coffee shops like Starbucks and Tim Hortons); pulling all-nighters when studying for an exam or preparing for an important presentation at work; not eating enough; and weather changes can send her mind into a tizzy.

Now what does she do to relieve the mental tension? She sometimes puts cold packs on her head; or retires early to sleep; but what doctors recommend and what most people do is lie in a very dark room with black out drapes so her eyes or brain are not exposed to light. And if the mental pain is too unbearable, she does take Tylenol to relieve some of the mental tension. During the several decades since she has had migraines no doctor has been able to help her. Same with my other friends and colleagues. Some are not even aware that lying in a darkened room will do the trick. I do recommend to you that if you are a sufferer of tension headaches or migraines, invest in some black out drapes in the room where you sleep, it will do wonders when a migraine strikes. If black out drapes are too costly and are not within your budget a great alternative would be to get a sleeping mask to cover your eyes from not much light getting to your brain.

Migraines, I should mention, affects more women than it does men for some reason. Actually, three times as much. Migraines affect about 3 million Canadians and up to one billion people worldwide, that's one-seventh of the world population. It's also the second most debilitating medical condition globally and more prevalent than diabetes and asthma combined.

Also, you may wish to cut down on your caffeine intake in soda, coffee, and tea as that might exacerbate your migraine.

I've had to impart the suggestion of the black out drapes to work colleagues who suffer from migraines who were in their forties and had never heard of that recommendation before. They were startled to know there was something additional they could do to help with their mental malady. I was glad I could pass that morsel of information I knew which they were grateful for.

As an addendum if you're suffering from migraines which cannot be remedied a good hospital to seek out is Women's College Hospital in Toronto, Canada, which has a Centre for Headaches. They see up to 5,000 patients annually who suffer from the condition.

Chapter 7
Constipation Relief

We, as humans, eat a lot of different kinds of foods. And if you live in a large American, Canadian, British, or some European country due to the influx of many immigrants there might be a whole plethora of different ethnic cuisines which you can order as take-out or visit a local restaurant to dine in. There are some cultures whose main staple in their diet could be rice-based. People from the Indian subcontinent, Caribbean countries, the Philippines, South Korea, Vietnam, Malaysia, and China do consume a lot of rice with their meals.

Rice is very glutenous and can lead to some people having constipation. It might be too hard to process within their bodies and not permit them to have good daily bowel movements, which is integral to having a good biological make-up.

I once worked with this woman of South Asian extraction who was from the country of Guyana. Mildred (not her real name) was beset with having daily constipation. This left her with feelings of discomfort and feeling bloated. Sure, she was still eating her three meals a day plus snacks but her persistent constipation was wreaking havoc with her health.

Mildred had seen several doctors and nothing they prescribed for her could alleviate the discomfort and lack of bowel movement she was experiencing. The thing was the doctors did not realize that she ate a lot of rice. That was the gist of her problem. Her daily lunch was always white rice with some side dish like curried meat or some vegetables.

It was only until I mentioned to her that she might want to cut back on the white rice was her problem solved. I conjecture her doctors failed to see that her daily consumption of white rice was the crux of the matter which led to her problem.

I also have a friend name Tracy whose mother is beset with the problem of constipation and by extension she too suffers from the same problem since they share the same DNA. Tracy and her Mom have tried flax seed, eating a lot of fiber, and using drugs like Senokot, but they don't seem to help all that much. Their problem is extreme. They don't want to use any laxatives like Exlax as they'd prefer not to infuse their bodies with too many drugs. If you're not aware, Senokot is a stool softener. I should mention it might take a day or so to work for those who would like to try it.

Also spreading flax seed in their foods did not work. But flax seed is good for anyone who has high cholesterol. It helps to lower the bad cholesterol in your system.

One thing which has worked like a charm for Tracy – who is Caucasian – is when she eats curried chicken. After an hour or so she always has a good bowel movement when all else fails. And she sometimes has an extreme case of constipation when she does not have a bowel movement for days. That being said, she, too, has tried Senokot, it works sometimes within a day or two on her system. But the extreme bloating, discomfort, and pain she feels is always relieved by her consuming curried chicken or some curried-based product.

Elderly people sometimes have extreme constipation. In seniors' homes they are sometimes given prune juice which works like magic for most of them. Or even consuming the fruit prune plum is just as good as drinking prune juice.

Adding more fiber to a person's diet could also work if the above options do not work for you if you suffer from constipation. There is not a one-size-fits-all solution when it comes to the nagging problem of constipation. And if you've ever suffered from this awful problem when there seems to be no solution you will try anything just to get relief.

If you suffer from this problem if might be good to add more fiber every day to your diet. Granola bars are another source of fiber just like Shreddies cereal. Be sure if you're taking eating a lot of fiber to be close to the washroom as you will never know when inspiration will strike. Brand buds may also work for others when other options fail or even trail mix. Nuts could be an excellent source of fiber. And stay away from gelatinous foods as they can be binding. Don't eat fruits which have not been ripen like green bananas as that will also bind you just like the aforesaid white rice. Those are only good if you have diarrhea as mentioned in a previous chapter.

Chapter 8
Lactose Intolerant

Humans were not really supposed to ingest cow's milk. Our ancestors who lived an agrarian lifestyle, where farming was the mainstay of their lives, and they subsisted on what they produced on the land, and also consumed the meats from farm animals like cows, chickens, ducks, goats, sheep, and pigs, including the milk from cows or goats, we as a people inherited that behavior from them. So, during the course of time into the Industrial Revolution and beyond we continued that habit and it became a daily part of our diet.

Over time our bodies either developed a tolerance or got acclimated to consuming dairy products like milk and its by-products like cheese, but we grew to love dairy products. Of course, with the advent of restaurants and diners in the fifties in America we also had other things added to the mix like delicious milk shakes.

But, one thing which began to occur – and we can develop this at any stage in life – is that some humans developed an intolerance to milk. What it is that humans become intolerant of is the lactose in milk. If as children we loved to drink milk and milk shakes and loved to eat grill cheese sandwiches, as we age either in our teens, twenties, thirties, forties, and beyond we may develop an intolerance to process lactose after we consume dairy products including yogurts as well. That being said, in some families it may be prevalent, but still some parents may not be lactose intolerant, but one or more of their children could be become lactose intolerant in childhood or as they get older.

Caucasians are the one ethnic group which have some members who are lactose intolerant but increasingly Asians, South Asians, and people of African descent. Some reports however peg that the issue is increasingly among Caucasians where other studies claim it's the opposite. In my years in the working world I have met many Caucasians who are lactose intolerant which defies what some of these studies claim. Keep in mind that some studies only use a sample group of a few thousands and the researchers make a conjecture from those findings. I've not read an exhaustive study in the hundreds of thousands of participants which corroborate these finds. Some doctors may also misdiagnose this condition among their patients when their patients may have some other underlying issued like gluten intolerance.

If dairy products seem to be an issue for you and they trigger things like bloating, diarrhea, or upset stomachs you could be a candidate for being lactose intolerant. Keep in mind, if you've never had the condition before it could develop with age. Our bodies change as we grow older. Even some foods we might like as children we may no longer have a palate for when older. Same goes with dairy products. You might have loved them as children but your body can no longer digest the lactose in the milk now that you're an adult.

But there is a saving grace. People with lactose intolerant – if they still enjoy drinking milk or having it in the morning coffee or tea – can use other substitutes which may taste just as good. Soy milk and almond milk are increasingly being used by people who are lactose intolerant. They have proved to be great substitutes for milk.

Some people however may be semi-lactose intolerant. Maybe they can't consume 2% milk but their bodies can still consume 1% or skim milk. I know some colleagues like that. They may not be able eat ice cream cones from ice cream trucks, but can still ingest sundaes from McDonald's cones, or even ice cream sandwiches they can purchase from a convenience store.

If you believe you have become lactose intolerant, I would urge you to get corroboration from your doctor. Your doctor could get an allergy test for you to see if, in fact, you are lactose intolerant. If you deduce that they might be wrong, seek a second, third, or even fourth opinion. No one doctor may have all the answers. I know from experience. One doctor told me I was lactose intolerant when I had some stomach issues at one stage of my life, he, however, was unequivocally incorrect. It was a stomach ailment which suddenly disappeared without any medical intervention. I had had a battery of tests and they all came back negative.

Chapter 9
Diabetes

Diabetes has become a growing problem in recent years. There are more and more people regardless of race who are becoming diabetic. Diabetes generally occurs when the pancreas is no longer able to produce insulin. There are two types of diabetes: Type 1 and Type 2. People who have Type 1 are classified as having this type if they are below 30 years of age; those with Type 2 are generally 30 or older. With the latter most people will be taking insulin. I have four people in my extended family who are Type 2 diabetics but none of them take insulin. They manage their condition by regulating their diet by watching what they eat on a daily basis. They also avoid foods with a high sugar content.

As disclosed to me by my family physician, if you are a diabetic it's still good to consume fruits and vegetables, in moderation, but avoid the ones with a high sugar content like grapes and watermelons, which have an excessive amount of sugar. Also avoid soft drinks which have on average 5 table spoons of sugar. If you must drink soft drinks go for the diet variety. Plus, still all those artificial sweeteners in soft drinks are not good for your body. Some artificial sweeteners can also be carcinogenic so research them if you choose to take them to see what you're putting in your body. I had one colleague who was consuming a lot of Diet Coke and it began to create bowel problems for him. Still, another diabetic who I know would get diarrhea from consuming too much Coke (in her pre-diabetic stage). She did not want to stop because she was addicted to the taste but the after effect was counterproductive to having a good start to her day.

For those who are diabetic, one of the things they could do, if they drink coffee and tea, they should substitute sugar in their beverage by adding one tea spoon of honey. They will not lose the flavor that natural sugars give. Also, brown sugar is not as potent as white sugar so that too could be a good alternative. If you are very brave you might want to get rid of adding sugar from your coffee or tea altogether. I have and I don't really see a difference. I only add brown sugar to my morning coffee but for the rest of the day, when I drink more coffee I do so sans sugar. I use to use honey but sometimes it would give me diarrhea. That being said, I had a boss who always added honey to her morning coffee because she was a borderline diabetic. Honey will not adversely affect most people. Some foods will affect some people but be totally innocuous to others.

People who normally live in the suburbs of a major city tend to sometimes have more issues when it comes to diabetes, hypertension (high blood pressure), and cholesterol. Again, I've not seen any exhaustive studies which tracks this phenomenon, so I will use my city to illustrate this, as I've read a number of studies which supports this theory pertaining to the city, I reside in.

In Toronto, the people who live in the 416-area code (that is the city proper) generally commute to work using public transit as it is usually quick, efficient, and less costly than driving. So, when these citizens depart for work or school every day they must walk to the bus stop, take the bus, then walk to the subway, or walk down stairs to the subway, or catch a second bus or streetcar, and then when they depart that vehicle they must walk to their office or factory. What all these people do is put in a lot of walking every day. Conversely, citizens who live in the 905-area code (that is the suburbs surrounding the city), they usually drive into work every day so they get little exercise walking. Most of their time is spent on highways or streets "sitting" in their cars. Ergo, they are getting little exercise. Those same people do a lot of sitting every day thereby not exercising their bodies. They are driving to and from work (or school if they are picking up their children, or if they are students in college or university), then when they get to their office or factory, they generally sit all day long. That leads to them gaining weight due to the lack of exercise.

In addition, those people who live in the 905-area code since they live in houses must drive every where they go: to the corner store, to the grocery store, to the mall, to the movie theater, to a restaurant etc. These people in the 905 due to them constantly sitting in their cars are getting very little exercise on a daily basis. A lot of them have excessive weight.

I have two friends who live in the 905-area code and who work in the eastern end of the city and downtown. They are of average build, but due to their excessive commute times, they order a lot of take-out food which is generally not that healthy or beneficial to their well-being.

Most of these people in the 905-area code due to their woeful lack of exercise have more incidences of diabetes, cholesterol, and high blood pressure. It's a fact compared to the ones who live in the city core and who do a lot of walking – which is exercise – every single day during their commute to and from work or school.

If you have diabetes it is possible to reverse it by changing your diet and getting more exercise. One famous person who has done this is the actor Halle Berry. She was diabetic and no longer is. There was another gentleman who I saw on the news, who was morbidly obese, and who was diabetic. He however was determined to change his lifestyle. He stopped eating junk food, started eating right, lost a lot of weight, and exercised every day. Voila! He is no longer diabetic.

I know of four people who are diabetic because their jobs entailed sitting all day long. The fifth member of their family is not diabetic because he walked every day, took public transit to and from work, and workouts on a daily basis. He has also cut down on his intake of sugar. Thus far, he has held off the condition which plagues his four other biological relatives. His grandmother died of diabetes complications and had also lost both of her legs due to having diabetes. I have a colleague right now who is going, unfortunately, blind due to complications attributed to diabetes. He never ate right, liked a lot of desserts, and never got any exercise for the vast majority of his life. Over the years he put on a lot of pounds. And, yes, he drove everywhere he went. So, in essence, he sat all day long, either in front of the TV or while in his SUV.

There are many factors which cause diabetes some of which I have already mentioned. They are age, weight, inactivity, race, and also pregnant women get something called gestational diabetes which generally goes away once she has given birth. The inactivity is a great factor because the body is generally sedentary all day when usually sitting at work or if a person is a couch potato at home parked in front of the TV.

If you get diabetes, it's not the end of the world. You can still live a relatively good life even if you have to take insulin. You will still have to watch what you eat but, rest assured, you can still have a good quality of life. When you change your diet at first it will be a chore, but like everything in life, it will become second nature, as you get more accustomed to it. We all have our crosses to bear and most people have their share of ailments that they must deal with. One recommendation I have for you is to read and learn more about your illness so you can better manage it, and even if you like things like alcohol, wine, beer, and a lot of desserts, there might be substitutes which might have less sugar content that you could consume. I have a relative who is diabetic but loves to eat Cinnabon every night. She loves the taste but all of the ones she eats are specifically for diabetics and have no sugar content.

But don't despair, you can still enjoy your life even with a condition like diabetes. Best of luck.

Chapter 10
Influenza, Pneumonia, and Bronchitis

Common colds have been a problem for humans for centuries. There is no known cure only remedies to make our symptoms more manageable and bearable. For some reason, men don't fair as well as women when they get a cold. It might have to do with biology or gender differences. A cold tends to strike men more harshly than women. Women can cope more easily. Maybe it's the way that Nature has hardwired the two different genders to cope with ailments. After all, childbirth is the hardest thing any human can go through and men don't have to bear that burden. Maybe Nature has programmed women with more coping mechanisms, since they have to carry a child for nine months prior to giving birth, and the process of giving birth is very painful for women.

There are remedies a person can take for a cold, most are over the counter medications like Tylenol or Advil, to help a person cope with a headache or lozenges to stem the tide if the cold is accompanied by a cough. There are other products which people swear by like NyQuil or Dayquil or NeoCitran. I swear by Swiss Herbal lozenges. They work really well for me when I have to suppress a cough at home, at work, or while I'm travelling on a crowded bus or subway during rush hour. Other people love Fishermen's Friend. Whatever lozenges work for you, are the best I would suggest, because as I've said before no two persons are alike, even if they are identical twins, because each might have their own traits.

When it comes to influenza (or more commonly known as the flu) that is more harsher than a cold. A person's body may ache, they are enervated or weakened, they may have headaches, they can't sleep, they might have runny noses, and they might have lost their appetite. Foods that they normally love they might have an aversion to. If their flu is accompanied with a cough the aforesaid lozenges will help to lessen their coughs. When they go to sleep at night it would be good to rub some Vicks VapoRub in their nostrils and on their neck. The VapoRub in their nostrils will cause a soothing vapor action in their throat and will prevent them from coughing too much. They should wrap a towel around their necks so as not to get the VapoRub on their sheets or pajamas (or whatever they may sleep in). Before they head out for work, if they are able to go to work, they should clean their nostrils of the Vicks VapoRub, and also clean it off their neck in the shower using a good amount of soap. Also, they should elevate their heads using a second pillow when sleeping at night. This will enable them to sleep and may not spur on a coughing fit as can sometimes happen when a person has a cough. They should never consume cold or warm milk before bed when they have the flu. That will cause phlegm in their throats and will cause them to cough when they retire to bed. I know from experience. After consuming milk when a person has a cough, they can have a coughing fit which last up to one hour. Yes, I know from experience. It would be pleasant for the person with the cough or for other members of their household who are trying to get to sleep.

And if your country or state or province gives free flu shots, I would urge you to get one. If you have a drug plan that permits you getting it, I would highly recommend it. It will not prevent the flu, but it will lessen the severity of it if you contract one of the strains that is prevalent that flu season. The flu shot is a great precaution because the flu or influenza kills 600,000 people annually worldwide (this figure is from 2018). And influenza does not discriminate. It kills old and young alike. Some people have claimed to get influenza after they received the flu shot, but that has never been proven as bona fide fact. It may be a fallacy, or the person who gets influenza after receiving the flu shot, may have already gotten a flu virus prior to getting the flu shot.

Pneumonia also is a silent killer. It also kills young and old alike. There are a few types of pneumonia: walking, viral pneumonia, and bacterial pneumonia. Viral pneumonia a person can contract from a virus; bacterial is contracted from bacteria left on things we all commonly use in our home or offices like sinks, door handles, elevator buttons, car doors, magazines in doctor's offices; and walking pneumonia is more milder in form where a person can still function and not have really severe symptoms that would keep them bed-ridden for days.

I've had pneumonia before. I will tell you how harrowing it feels. You will be unable to sleep at night; even if you're wearing two layers of clothes and the heat is turned up, you will feel that it is twice as cold as it is; and when you cough because your lungs are filled with liquid, you will feel the sensation of drowning. It is not pleasant at all. And some nights you will not be able to sleep and might cough through the entire night. There are two types of pneumonia shots you can get, one which lasts five years and you will have to get it every five years, and another which you will only have to get once. I've had the former one 3 times. **Pneumovax** you will only have to get once and it covers 23 strains of the pneumonia bacteria. The pneumococcal bacteria can cause things like blood infections, lung infections, or even meningitis. Just as a word of caution: the third time I got the pneumonia shot (the one which lasts five years), the day after there was some redness on my arm and chess and stiffness in my arm. I had never experienced this side effect before. Thankfully about three days after, the side effect went away. The second type called **Pneumovax** costs over $100 and can prevent up to 23 different types of pneumococci bacteria as mentioned above. If you can afford it, and you've had pneumonia before, it just might save your life. So, I would consider getting it soon. I will when my person funds allow. I never want to be sick with pneumonia again as I've always said "it is the only form of legal torture."

Bronchitis is when a person has an infection of the bronchial tubes which is by your throat. It can cause tremendous coughing. Most people can still function when they have bronchitis, but some may be so enervated or weaken, that they will have to stay home from work or school. Some people with bronchitis even with their coughing can still go to work. Bronchitis is not contagious. A person can get medication prescribed by a doctor or take over the counter medications like Tylenol or Advil or lozenges to lessen their symptoms.

A had a former co-worker who got bronchitis a few times when I worked with her. She coughed all day long within the vicinity of me, and our other coworkers, but not one of us ever caught her bronchitis. She mainly had a dry cough and often had coughing spasms.

I once had bronchitis but I was weakened and had to stay home from work. It was mixed with symptoms of influenza. Although I had energy and could sleep at night, I was still felt enervated. I suspect I also had flu-like symptoms coupled with the bronchitis. My bronchitis took 3 weeks to run its course. A lady I took the bus with some mornings also had bronchitis. She coughed during our ten-minute ride to the subway in the morning seated beside me on the bus, and I never caught it from her.

Some things to do to prevent yourself from getting influenza, a cold, pneumonia, or bronchitis: wash your hands during flu seasons because you will often touch bus or subway poles, door knobs at work or at home, elevator buttons, shopping carts, that other people have touched; get enough sleep because when your body gets insufficient rest your immunity is not as strong; eat right and don't miss a meal; if you get a cold or cough, when you do cough do so in the crevice of your arm (some people still cough in their hands and then shake other peoples hands thereby passing on their germs – if I have a cold or cough, I inform people why I will not shake their hands or hug them); don't kiss your spouse, friends, or loved ones if you have a cold, cough, or flu, you'll just be passing on your germs (my wife's family still kisses each other when they're sick and their ailment is just passed around, my birth family does not); and get enough exercise. These may be simple measures, but people tend to forget some of these simple steps when we approach and head into flu season every year. Yes, they are simple but they do work.

(As an addendum: some people might be carriers of the flu virus but not manifest the symptoms themselves. But they can still pass on the virus. These people are called Typhoid Mary. It is named after an Irish domestic worker who passed on typhoid fever but never actually got typhoid fever herself. She infected about 51 people while working as a cook. So, some people can be carriers but still remain immune to the disease they are carrying.)

Chapter 11
Sleep an Elixir

We all need an adequate amount of sleep every night. When a person does not get a sufficient amount of sleep when they lay down to rest at night it can adversely affect their health. It can make their day at work fraught with stress, making bad indecisions, costly mistakes, and them being curt with people they work with. It can cause them to be very irritable as well. There are some vocations where the workers need to get a good amount of sleep every night. Those vocations include jobs like surgeons, nurses, police, emergency workers, air traffic controllers, pilots, people using heavy or dangerous machinery, driving buses or trains, and fire fighters. If the decisions you make on your job can have a perilous effect on those you deal with, having enough sleep is paramount. **A good suggestion that most medical experts agree with is to have at least 7 to 8 hours of sleep per night. That will enable a person to have a good clarity of mind when on the job.**

One colleague had a doctor who encouraged her to have at least 10 hours of sleep per night. I have another colleague who insisted on getting 9 hours of sleep per night. I have to admit the few nights when I can get 10 hours of sleep, I feel invincible during the course of the day. There are some people who cannot sleep very much per night. I had a former colleague who only received 4 hours of shut-eye per night. Guess what? She was often times very irritable. Her internal biology clock would only permit her to sleep for 4 hours. She did get in a lot of reading done during the time she was up and her family was getting their 7 or 8 hours however. I have to admit the few times in my life when I have had insomnia, I have felt extremely tired during the course of the day, and when I returned home from work, I usually went straight to bed for a 1 or 2 hour nap which help to alleviate the lack of sleep somewhat. My body would feel totally enervated and like lead on some of those days. I fear not getting enough sleep.

Some things a person should do to get their requisite 7 or 8 hours per night is to not have caffeine close to bed. Some doctors say don't have it after 3pm others say don't have it after 5pm or 7pm. Office workers are said to experience the 3pm hump. That is when their bodies start to feel sluggish and lethargic and they need a burst of energy from coffee, tea, or some soda which has caffeine.

When I worked for a medical company it was usually around 3pm when I started to feel sluggish some days. Fortunately, we had good-tasting free coffee in the office. I would always have a cup to give me that jolt of energy and then head back to my desk to finish my day's work. It served me well and I was able to function optimally for the remainder of the day. Some of my former co-workers would have up to 5 cups of coffee per day and could still sleep at night which I found astounding. If I have more than 3 cups per day, I will be up all night staring at the ceiling. That being said, also if I have tea or coffee after 8pm, I also will be up all night usually until 2am just tossing and turning. I however would try to gauge how best you can handle caffeine as everyone is not built the same.

Also, it would be a good rule of thumb not to exercise too close to bed. The adrenaline will be flowing through your body and that will keep you up as well. Some people (like myself) do a light workout in the evening and can still sleep every night like a baby. I usually do a light workout while watching the 10pm news. I've been doing it for 32 years and it has not impeded my ability to sleep.

Don't read an eBook or use your cellphone close to bed. The light from either one will filter into your brain and keep it active thereby preventing you from sleep. Staring at light is not conducive to getting a good night's sleep. Researchers have found that young people using their cellphones too close to bedtime has prevented them from having good shut-eye every night. And teenagers in high school and young adults in college or university do need as much sleep as they can get.

Sleep is like an elixir. The body really needs its rest every night. That is how humans and animals are programmed. Sleep lets us program our minds and gives us rest from the mental toxins of the day. Having a good night's sleep will help a person make a good decision in the morning. You may notice that if you're mulling over a problem, or if you're an executive who has to make an important decision, getting enough sleep will give you the clarity of mind to do so the next day. Your mind also processes the information you mentally intake during the day when you sleep. Ever notice that something you may have read, or studied just before you got to bed, you remember with great clarity when you wake up in the morning? There have been some great discoveries which have benefited humankind which were made by intelligent people while they slept. Sting, the musician, actually has gotten out of bed to write down a song that was entering his subconscious as he was either sleeping or drifting off to sleep. The mind is a mysterious thing. It's very active and we must learn to tame it and control it. And sleep permits us to do so.

Sleep also enables us to fight off diseases and ailments. When we are sick, we need as much sleep as we can get. The body and mind heal better when we are sleeping. Sleep is a great regenerative tool that God has given us to better enable us to deal with diseases and sickness.

If you would like to tire the mind and prepare yourself to sleep, drink a warm glass of milk which you can heat in the microwave. It will enable you to have a restful night. (However, remember if you are sick with a cough or the flu, having a glass of warm milk will cause phlegm, prompting you to cough preventing you from sleeping.) But don't forget to brush your teeth before bed as you don't want the milk to sit on your teeth and cause tooth decay. You can also read a book or a magazine or newspaper in hardcopy before you go to bed. That will tire out your mind and let you drift into the unconscious. Never have an argument before bed as that will keep you up. Deal with your issue or problem in the morning. Having a warm bath or shower might also help you get into the mood of sleeping. Some have claimed that making love also tires them out and causes the body to feel relieved which prepares them for bed. Sometimes sexual tension can keep your mind racing preventing you from sleeping. If you're a writer, try not to write too close to bed as that will cause your mind to work overtime, and your active mind may prevent your from falling asleep. Your mind might continue to race with ideas when you retire to your bed. But remember to get your 7 or 8 hours of shut-eye every night then you will be well equipped to start the next day refreshed and recharged. Researches have also recently discovered – which is not really a great revelation – that the people who get an adequate amount of sleep per night tend to be more optimistic. That's another reason to get enough sleep: your glass will always be half full and you might also have a sunny disposition. Some plane crashes and major industrial accidents have occurred because the pilots or people running the equipment like a large ship were lacking in sleep. The more sleep you get; the better your performance will be either on the job, or if you're still pursuing your studies in college or university, or if you have to make a very important presentation to your staff, or a large group of people like at a convention, or symposium.

Chapter 12
Walking and Exercise

Our human ancestors were nomads always hunting for their food or foraging for their next meal. Humans tend to be more sedentary either sitting in their office or factory jobs doing the same routine task day in and day out. All this sitting has left us susceptible to possibly colon cancer. That coupled with bad diets does not bode well for our long-term health. However, we can do something to remedy that. What can we do? We can try to get more exercise!

Every year on New Year's Eve one of the resolutions that most people make is to get more exercise. That's a noble idea but most start by getting a gym membership and then they fall off the wagon. There is a rush for gym memberships in January every year but by March most people stop going to the gym. It happens every year.

You can still get exercise on your way to work. If you take a bus to subway, why not walk those few blocks to the subway, especially if the weather is nice? Or on your way home why don't you walk those same few blocks back home?

You could purchase a bicycle with a helmet and elbow pads and go riding around your neighborhood. I know riding to and from work may be a problem for some people due to distance, but also competing with cars especially when you have cars who will not yield to cyclists. That could make riding perilous for cyclists. In some major cities – especially in Europe and some parts of North America – there are streets with designated bike lanes which is great! Before China before more industrialized, the Chinese rode everywhere. That is why when you see older pictures of people in China, they are all so thin and physically fit. Now that there is more affluence in China everyone drives everywhere, ergo, they are losing the exercise they use to get by riding their bicycles to and from work.

If you like walking, you could get a walking buddy and go walking around your neighborhood after dinner. That surely will add to the amount of exercise you get every day. If you want to track the number of steps you get every day, buy a cheap pedometer, which will count the number of steps you do every day. The pedometer does not have to be expensive, there are very cheap ones on the market. Doctors recommend that a person should try to at least get 10,000 steps in every day. That's a noble goal to pursue. Also, if you will be using the subway, and have no mobility issues, go up or down the stairs at the subway. There is no need to take the elevator if you're an able-bodied person.

If you live in a condominium or apartment why not go up and down the stairs in your building when you leave for work and when you arrive home? That will add to the amount exercise you're getting and will no doubt make you feel better. You will also be able to get a good night's sleep.

Of while you're watching the nightly news, you should use some free weights – they don't have to be really heavy – maybe 5, 10, or 15 lbs. depending on what you're able to handle. Also add some sit-ups to the mix. That may lower your waste line and also make you feel better. Truth be known a large waste line could lead to heart problems later. Men who drink beer sometimes get a "beer gut," or who sit down all day at work (whether behind a desk or while driving a truck, taxi, or if they are a sales person driving to and from appointments). After work they also probably drive home and again are sitting in their cars or SUVs. They consume a lot of calories at breakfast, lunch, and dinner but do not get any exercise. They may also consume a bottle of beer after dinner which is not a good thing when it comes to maintaining a good waist line.

When you start your exercise regimen, you can start with little increments and then work your way up. You don't have to aim for a body like Arnold Schwarzenegger in his prime, you just want to get a good cardiovascular workout to benefit your heart. You need a good heart to last you a lifetime. And if you smoke, you might want to ditch the habit as that can lead to a stroke. I've had two former colleagues who were avid smokers and who both had strokes. The former recovered but the second did not. She is still using a walker four years after her stroke. They both fortunately did quit smoking after their strokes. I also have a neighbor who had a mild heart attack – she is also a very avid smoker – she has had some stents put into her arms, but she, unfortunately, has not given up smoking. She also still has the worst and very harsh-sounding smoker's cough. I'm sorry to say that some people will learn the hard way. I wish her well.

Or even if you can join a softball, ball hockey, volleyball, tennis, or basketball league for amateurs that will enable you to get some exercise because I'm sure your job entails sitting all day. Even people who don't work in offices do a lot of sitting all day. Bus drivers, gas station attendants, convenience store clerks, retail workers, etc. all do a lot of sitting during the course of their busy days.

Whatever exercise you can get in during the day, that will benefit no one but you in the end, so get a move on! You will thank yourself later.

Chapter 13
Dementia

Dementia has become a growing issue amongst the elderly of our population. Some people are getting dementia which can also be interchangeably mixed in with Alzheimer's at an alarming early age. Some are showing signs of it at a very early age. The adult brain starts to show signs of mild memory loss around the age of 40. As we approach and get into our fifties it is becoming more pronounced in some of our population. **Dementia and Alzheimer's are mainly caused by the mind not purging the amyloid beta which accumulates during the day as we go about our daily business.** It's like plaque forming on the brain. When we sleep our minds are purged of the amyloid beta giving us a much more clearer minds when we awake in the morning. That's why sleep is very beneficial to the human mind. That being said, there are some adults who live into their eighties and their nineties and still have very sharp minds. Just yesterday I saw a lady on the news who was 101 years old and her mind was sharp as a tact. God bless her.

There were two adults in my wife's maternal and paternal extended families who lived into their nineties and their minds were still very clear. Their level of cognition was better than some people in their twenties. One thing these two of my wife's relatives did was read every day. They always read a daily newspaper and always had a book on the go as well. My wife also has two elderly friends of the family – Beverly and Esther (not related to each other) – who are well into their eighties and still have very sharp memories. Beverly worked until a few years ago until she was about 86 and Esther is still working at that age. She likes to get out of the house to keep her mind and body very active. Beverly had to quit working as she had many ailments one being kyphosis, which is a curvature of the spine, typically referred to as a hump back. But still Beverly drives her car and gets around quite easily.

My wife's paternal aunt Mary lived until she was 90 years of age. Her mind was very clear right until the end of her life. She read the newspaper every day and always had a book on the go as well. Her maternal uncle Murray, is still going strong at 90 years of age. He owns a business, and still checks in on it every so often, but has largely left the day to day operation of it to his two sons. Murray starts his day by reading two newspapers to keep abreast of what is happening locally in his city, the nation, and the world.

I once had a boss who was age 55. He was a nice man but at that early age was showing signs of dementia. He read every day and kept trying to learn new things. He also knew how to write some computer code. He had a university degree and started his own business which was going strong for 25 years. His name was Craig and his mind was faltering.

I sat beside Craig in the same office for five months. He would continually tell me the same stories about work and his personal life over and over and over again. It was like a non-stop loop that would not stop. One day he would impart some anecdote about his life, and then the next day would recount the story he just told me the day before. I would indulge him and let him tell the story as I knew it gave him a modicum of pleasure to relive that moment in his life. Craig, however, was well aware that his mind was slowly fading away. Craig was the vice-president of the company. He would also have conference calls with the company's biggest client every Tuesday. It was disheartening for me, but he was constantly recounting the same stories to his clients on the phone. They were men in their thirties so I know Craig's clients on the other line could recognize that he was suffering from some sort of dementia. Our department would also have weekly meetings. It was Craig, two female coworkers (one who was 24 and the other was 30 years of age), and myself. Craig, again, would recount the same stories over and over and over again. I would look at the faces of my two female coworkers with the recognition that Craig had told these anecdotes – which he often did at the end of our meetings – that he was telling these stories for the umpteenth time. I felt like telling Craig's wife, who was the accountant in the office, but I did not want to upset the apple cart. Craig needed medication and fast.

He had imparted to me once in private that he knew his memory was fading.

I have a male biological relative who's in his seventies who is also suffering from the early stages of dementia. He is however getting some treatment and is going to some programs to help him with his condition. He tries to keep active by gardening and going for walks every day. He also has a nap every day which I think is helping to keep his dementia at bay.

My mother-in-law is suffering from the same condition. She's is about 86 right now and her mind is rapidly fading. She has been suffering from it for about seven or eight months now and she can't recall almost anything. She forgets something that transpired 5 minutes ago, that's how bad her memory has gotten. And her long-term memory she is obscured meaning that what she recalls about it is not, in fact, based in reality. Those events never occurred. She's almost been reduced to the mindset of a child. She has PSWs (Personal Support Workers) who come in three times a week to take care of her and to give my father-in-law some respite from taking care of her. My wife has been doing a lot of heaving lifting, as she visits her mother regularly, and takes over lunch for her about three times a week. My wife is an angel. As are the PSWs.

More women, for some reason, suffer from dementia or Alzheimer's than men. A Canadian statistic pegs it at about 61% of suffers of dementia are female. And about 2/3 of caregivers from families are female who take care of their elderly relative who is suffering from this black dog of the mind.

Over the 20 years of my marriage with my beloved wife I have been exposed to a lot of elderly friends of her parents. A lot of them are blessed with sharp minds. Why? I have observed that all the ones with who read every day have really great mental cognition into their eighties. They all have great memories and are repositories of so much great information. They are all walking history books. Most of them usually read the newspaper every day and also continually have a book they are reading. They also have a very active social life and like to keep busy. My wife's aunt Fey who died in her early eighties read three books every week which she would get from the library. She always said her mind was "very sharp." Before she died her last words to me was "love each other." Auntie Fey was a gem as are her other elderly relatives and her parents and their friends.

So, what you can you do as a person do to stave off dementia? For one, exercise your mind every day. The most important thing you can do is read. Socialize. Socializing with friends keep you connected and you form a bond which is mutually beneficial with others. If you have the monetary means you should travel. Or if you own a car go for short drives or explore your city using public transit. Gardening is also a good activity that keeps your body and mind engaged. If you're the creative type maybe you should journal, sketch, or paint with watercolors. If you have musical talent try practicing your instrument every day. Write letters to friends or relatives, I'm sure they would like to receive a letter in the mail. Or if you prefer type them an email. (My mother is in her seventies and she texts her grandchildren, my wife, her children, and her siblings in the United States every day. She also likes to do Word Search games every day in a hard copy book, or play Candy Crush or Tetris on her iPad. It's keeping her mind active during her golden years.) Do crosswords or Sudoku or word search games yourself. Go see a movie with a friend. Or why not go out with your neighbor or a friend for coffee. It's inexpensive and you can both catch up on what is happening in each other's lives. There are days when the senior's price for a movie ticket is less than other days, so those are the days you might wish to see a movie, as most seniors are on fixed incomes. Go for a walk every day. Having an active body means having an active mind. I live next to a seniors' residence most of whom are in their eighties or nineties. And most of those seniors go for a walk down the block every day even if they use walkers. If you knit keep up the hobby as that will keep your mind active as well. If you like the theater go a see a play. Wednesday or Saturday matinees are usually cheaper and you will still see a great play. Look for free performances in your city as there are some production companies which offer PWYC (pay-what-you-can) for summer productions. Or get a part-time job or volunteer at your local soup kitchen, hospital, or food bank, I'm sure they could use the help. There was a gentleman in his seventies who worked in the call center in the last company I was employed at. He did a good job due to his many years of experience. There was another senior who worked for our call center but who worked from home. There is a retired gentleman who lives in my condo building who still drives a school bus, takes tap dancing lessons, and has joined a gym which he visits every day. He also took a European vacation this past summer.

But whatever you do to keep your mind active, keep doing it. Don't just sit home watching TV and being a couch potato. That's the worst thing you could possibly do to stave off dementia. An active person means they have an active mind and body. Like the old adage goes: use it or lose it!

Chapter 14
Cold Sores

Cold sores have plagued some of us since we were in elementary school. I know it has afflicted me since I was in grade five. And, believe me, it's not good at all when they sprout up like mushrooms on the sides of your lip. Cold sores are part of the herpes virus. I surmise mine might have surfaced because I started to kiss my girlfriends at a very early age and they may have given it to me. But I'm not complaining, they were my girlfriends, they meant no harm, and I enjoyed kissing them because after all it was puppy love.

Cold sores can sometimes last a few days, or for the unfortunate few of us, can last a week or more. Once when I had the flu, cold sores broke out on both sides of my mouth and they really grew large. Thankfully, at the time, the young lady with whom I took the bus with to work, did not look at me like I had some awful communicable disease. She just took it in stride and did not have a scornful look on her face when she looked at my awful cold sores.

I believe it was a doctor who told me this remedy when I was a child. He told me to sterilize a bobby pin under hot water for several minutes and then pierce my cold sores as soon as I felt them appearing. **Remember if you choose this method you must sterilize the bobby pin under scalding hot water from your tap. Don't do it on the stove as you might burn yourself.** Scalding hot water from your tap will suffice.

This method has served me well since I was in grade five and I am now in middle age. I would then put some Vaseline on it and it usually gets better within a few days. The odd time there will be a crust that forms which will fall off in due time and not leave a scar. Remember when you use the bobby pin, after sterilizing it with hot water, to also get a Kleenex tissue to collect the blood or the liquid that will be seeping out. Just swab it gently with the Kleenex tissue. And remember to discard the tissue when done. Don't reuse it. Keep doing this until the blood and liquid stops coming out. Then apply the Vaseline. Most people who I suggest to use this method must think I'm crazy. But it's worked for me for over 40 years.

There are some people who swear by the product Abreva. This product is a cold sore cream and is sold over the counter at drug stores. I've never used it but my father-in-law swears by it. As soon as he gets a cold sore, he runs to the drug store to get it. It might work for you too if you choose not to use the sterilized needle method.

Also, one word of caution. If you have a cold sore, don't participate in oral sex. I have a male friend who had a girlfriend perform fellatio on him while she had a cold sore. Wrong move! This occurred when he was in his early twenties and ever since he has flair ups of cold sores on his penis. So, before careful. Even if you're a man, don't perform cunnilingus on your female partner if you have a cold sore. That will lead to her also getting a sexually transmitted disease and to much pain for her. In short, oral sex is a very risky way to have sex.

Just to protect both you and your partner, if you will be performing cunnilingus, please use something that will inhabit you from touching the clitoris directly. I would suggest you use some Saran Wrap or a female condom which is sold in drugstores. This will also prevent either of you from getting oral cancer in the event your partner has the HPV (Human Papilloma Virus) or you can give her sores by her clitoris. Be safe, then there will be no lifelong regrets for either of you.

Chapter 15
Carpal Tunnel Syndrome

Carpal tunnel syndrome or repetitive strain injury is a scourge of modern-day offices. Most office workers spend their day at computers either typing out documents, entering some sort of date, writing emails, working on spreadsheets, or using Power Point. A lot of these tasks involve the repetitive motion of the hands typing on their QWERTY keyboards or entering numbers as well. This involves a lot of the same motions done hundreds of times even thousands of times each day. Over a year or years this can lead to the carpal tunnel in the wrist being damaged.

I have had some friends and coworkers who work in offices either had to have surgery on their wrists – which alleviated some of the pain they were feeling but did not cure their condition – or had cortisone shots in their wrists. The latter can be very painful and can leave them feeling limb-wristed with a lot of discomfort the day after receiving the needles. Not something I would wish on my worst enemy. There is even a colleague I've had who has had the surgery on her carpal tunnel which rendered her unable to work following the surgery. That was not a good outcome.

I have devised a great remedy which can help with this condition. It was not taught to be any therapists or doctor, I just logically thought of what we do when we type and, in the process tried to rectify this condition. Doctors have not really come up with a salient treatment for carpal tunnel syndrome besides surgery. That however is also very painful and will leave scars and not really rectify the problem. My treatment is non-invasive, and I've told a few colleagues with whom I've worked, who suffer from shoulder issues as well as carpal tunnel syndrome, due to all the typing they do at their jobs, day in and day out.

The first part of this treatment involves using light weights. After work every night a person should do wrist curls with 5 lbs. or 10 lbs. weights. For women I would recommend they use the 5 lbs. weights and men should use the 10 lbs. weights. First start off with 10 wrist curls then graduate to 20, 30, 40, 50 repetitions until they reach 100. You should do them rapidly not slowly. If you do them slowly you will hurt your wrist. Then continue doing those 100-wrist curls every night. The motion basically is lifting the weight only using your wrist. Because our wrists are delicate this will strengthen the carpal tunnel in your wrists. Ergo, you will feel less pain when you type. You could do the repetitions while watching TV. I've been doing 100 repetitions (on each wrist) for 25 years every night while watching the nightly news. It just takes me 5 minutes total for both wrists. This strengthens my carpal tunnel and my forearm. Biologically women have more delicate forearms and wrists than men. This method will work for both females and males.

The second part of this treatment is to act shrewdly when you're using a Word document or Excel spreadsheet or email. Don't use your mouse to scroll up and down the screen!!! Instead there is a bar on the right side of your screen when you're in a Word

doc, or Excel spreadsheet, or email. Use your mouse to drag down the page if need be by using that bar. By using your mouse to scroll through the document you're putting undue strain on your wrists which will exacerbate your condition and make it worst day by day. These methods have worked for me exceedingly well when no doctor could help me.

I have used these two methods every day for close to 25 years and they have served me well. No more trips to the doctor because all they propose are band-aid solutions without addressing the problem at its root. That is, what is actually causing the problem, and how can a person rectify what they are doing to not cause the problem in the first place. I've sat in one ergonomics seminar to teach me better habits at work and not once did the person conducting the seminar address the issue about how to rectify carpal tunnel syndrome. All they did was talk about your posture, how you're sitting in relation to your screen, is your foot firmly on the ground, or are you slouching. All these do not address the problem directly.

If you use my easy and logical methods, they will save you undue pain in your wrists, and also will avoid you having to get surgery which will not fix the problem. I would also advise you to ask your employer for a light touch keyboard. Or, if you work from home, get a light touch keyboard as typing on a keyboard where you have to strike the keys very hard will put needless pressure on your wrist. But I surmise most computers today come with light touch keyboards – all the better for people who sit at a computer for most of their working day. Most, if not all laptops, have keyboards which are light touch.

Chapter 16
Oral Health

Our oral health is one of the most important aspects for our well-being as it affects our entire body. If we are not taught good oral hygiene when we are children, we will not tend to practice good oral hygiene when we get older. I have worked with some individuals who sometimes don't brush their teeth in the morning. There was one person who never bothered to brush her teeth at all. There was a lot of foreign things in her mouth and her breath was malodorous. To say the least being her vicinity to have a conversation was very challenging.

If we don't practice good oral hygiene that can lead to tooth decay and eventually the lost of a tooth or teeth as we get older. And, of course, we need our teeth for life.

I marvel when I see a centenarian on the news who has all their own teeth. Those people are magical.

There is an excellent quote which I gleaned from an op-ed in the newspaper written by Dr. Hazel Stewart, who is the former director for dental and oral health for the City of Toronto, and here's how a portion of it reads: **"Scientific evidence suggests that having an unhealthy mouth could be contributing to chronic diseases of the heart, lung and stomach as well as being a risk factor for diabetes. The effects of chronic poor oral health can be physically debilitating and socially incapacitating. It can affect a person's ability to eat healthy foods, to sleep, to work and to maintain social connections."** Which basically says it is of paramount importance to have good oral health as without it, bad oral health adversely affects our entire existent in various aspects.

Having excellent oral health can also affect our organs and our blood stream as well.

There were some coworkers who I've worked with who were the best at taking care of their oral health. They would brush after the lunch every day and it showed.

Their teeth and mouths were always clean and they never had bad breath. There was one gentleman who drank several cups of coffee every day to keep his energy and alertness on the job. By the afternoon he was in the washroom brushing his teeth around 2pm or 3pm. He consumed maybe about 3 or 4 cups of coffee per day. There were others though who consumed up to 5 cups of coffee and did not brush their teeth. This showed on the discoloration of their teeth and their halitosis due to their tongues being dry, which is not a good thing, especially when you are in close quarters with other people every day, and closely interacting with them.

There was one lady whose halitosis was so bad you could smell it from at least six feet away. People stayed far away from her when they conversed with her. Believe me, it was not a pleasant experience. Practicing good oral hygiene can also help with your romantic relationships especially if you have a steady boyfriend or girlfriend or are lawfully wedded.

Some things we should do to maintain excellent oral hygiene is brush at least twice a day: in the morning before we start our day and at night before we go to sleep. If we don't brush before we go to sleep, we will have food remnants, and the sugars from alcohol or beverages or juices we consumed during the day sitting on our teeth, which can ultimately lead to tooth decay, which is one of the worst things we can do for ourselves.

I, personally, brush my teeth 3 times a day. In the morning, after I get home from work, and before I go to sleep. If I have a nap, I also do a little brush when I awake so that would amount to 4 times some days.

A person should also floss before bed to clear any food deposits between their teeth. Most people are reluctant to do this and only have their teeth flossed when they go to a dental hygienist. Anyone should do it before they see a dental hygienist and practice flossing every day. Brushing alone will not clean our teeth to the nth degree.

Also replace your toothbrush once every few weeks. A toothbrush with a lot of splay bristles is not doing the job it is supposed to. And don't get a tooth brush with hard bristles as that is bad for your gums. Get one with medium or soft bristles. And whatever you do, don't share your toothbrush with your spouse or romantic partner. Yes, I know you must French kiss and do open mouth kissing. All our toothbrushes have germs on them. The human mouth is one of the filthiest places due to all the different kinds of foods we eat. It has been said that a dog's mouth is much cleaner than a human's. The reason being is that humans consume a lot of different foods whereas a dog only generally eats one type or two types of food. Yes, there is the prospect that some dogs groom themselves in their rear nether regions but, it has been said, that a dog's mouth is still cleaner than a human's.

Also, if you're really steadfast about having a really clean mouth, you might want to augment your flossing by using tooth picks in those really hard to reach places. There are some people who have never gotten their wisdom teeth extracted so using tooth picks might help in those cases.

To also circumvent getting halitosis (or bad breath) we should brush our tongues. Use a toothbrush with soft bristles and moisturize our tongues in the morning and before going to sleep at night. There are a lot of people who don't do this and it can lead to halitosis. However, halitosis sometimes cannot be cured with just by brushing the tongue, as for some people it might stem to some stomach issues or glandular issues, and the person might have to see a specialist. That being said, breath mints only mask the problem of halitosis, in most cases by brushing your tongue that might alleviate the problem. Our tongues you might notice after you awake in the morning is generally covered in a white film of debris. That needs to be scraped off with your tooth brush. At first you might not like the sensation of brushing your tongue, but you will get use to it in time, and it will do you a world of good.

So, practice good oral health, and you might be making less trips to the dentist for things like cavities, crowns, or those dreaded root canals. Since I have practiced excellent oral health for most of my life, I have not had a cavity since I was 10 years old, and I am now in middle age. Knock wood – I hope I have to never get another one for the rest of my life. And I hope the same for you too.

In addition to the above suggestion I would implore you to rinse right after you consume, beer, wine, alcohol, chips, candies, or chocolate. All that sugar sitting on your teeth is bad for your teeth and can also lead to tooth decay. And the teeth whiteners you find in drug stores are mostly bad for whitening your teeth as most of them destroy the enamel on your teeth. It would be best to see a dentist who could whiten your teeth much more safely and not destroy your enamel in the process. Most dentists will produce a mould of your teeth just in case you need to return for further whitening down the road. I had a co-worker whose uncle was a dentist and she had the best-looking teeth. Also, when you consume wine, beer, alcohol, tea, coffee, or sugary sodas, always use a straw to drink your beverage. This way the liquid bypasses your teeth and goes directly to your throat. With plastic straws becoming slowly obsolete I would suggest using a paper or metal straw. The former is environmentally-friendly and the latter is reusable.

I should mention there was one work colleague I worked with when I was in my twenties. While a few of my coworkers and I were having lunch one day we started to discuss tooth fillings. To our astonishment, our colleague Rosanna did not have one single filling. She had gone through childhood, adolescences, and was in her mid-twenties and never once had her mouth ever seen a dentist's drill. We were all amazed. She also had nice white straight teeth. Her smile was also very nice. We are all mightily impressed.

Practice good oral hygiene. It will be good for your health and you will also make less trips to the dentist's chair. In closing, you might wish to use some mouthwash like **Listerine**. Having said that, just pouring out the Listerine liquid may be harsh on your gums. I would suggest you dilute it with water before rinsing and then it will be less harsh on your gums. But, on the plus side you will have great smelling breath and people will love to be around you. I would suggest you use 50% Listerine and 50% water in the cap from the bottle for a quick rinse every morning or before bed. **Oral Rinse** is also good to use and again should be diluted with the same ratio as mentioned above. And don't forget to get your teeth cleaned by a dental hygienist every 6 months. If your work has a dental plan, by all means, make use of it. You will save a lot of money and your oral health will be better for it. You need your teeth for life!

Chapter 17
Taking Aspirin, Does it Help?

It has been a long-held belief that taking a daily Aspirin will help to stave off a heart attack. That has been refuted in recent years. However, people swear that taking a daily Aspirin can help in the event of a heart attack. In fact, I have a colleague who does just that. The reason being his father died of a heart attack and he thinks by consuming an Aspirin every day will help in the event he has one.

I also have a relative who takes an Aspirin every day but that is because he has had two heart attacks. That's what doctors now recommend. **A daily Aspirin will not help anyone to stave off a heart attack, it's just those individuals who have already had one. That is now the common medical belief.**

Also, now when a person experiences a heart attack, that is what a paramedic will give the person when they pick, he or she up, before taking them to the hospital. A paramedic will give that person an Aspirin to chew on. By taking an Aspirin that will increase the blood flood to the heart and avoids clumping therefore preventing a heart attack. Chewing on an Aspiring will increase blood flow to the heart thereby assisting the person from having further damage to the heart if the person is having a coronary attack.

Some have claimed that a daily Aspirin will also help in preventing cancer and getting dementia. These two other benefits of Aspirin are not wildly known. Taking low dosages of Aspirin (that is, baby Aspirin) is said to also lower blood pressure if taken at bed time. It can also help in the event of a stroke by preventing blockages.

Keep in mind, a heart attack can be misdiagnosed by medical professionals. Even cardiologists. Some may not even see the signs. For example, my father-in-law was complaining for three days or more of chest pains. He said it felt like someone was sitting on his chest. He went to the emergency department of two hospitals, one which is very renowned in my city, and they said he had nothing to worry about. He also saw an eminent cardiologist, who also told him there was nothing to worry about, after he had seen my father-in-law's x-rays.

Still days after, my father-in-law kept complaining of chest pains and this "weight on his chest." When he still could not take it any longer, he called for an ambulance and was taken to a third or fourth hospital. There the medical staff were finally able to deduced that he, in fact, was having a heart attack. He, subsequently, spent a week in that hospital until he recovered. So, you see a heart attack cannot be diagnosed by some of the best doctors.

My colleague, whose father died of his heart attack, made it to the hospital but, unfortunately, his father succumbed to his heart attack. He woke up on a Monday morning and complained of chest pains. He brushed his teeth then went to a hospital. He died shortly after.

Another relative has a had two and he has had stents put into the arteries in in his thigh to prevent further blockages. Stents are these little mesh-like devices which are placed into your arteries to prevent any blockages.

My elderly neighbor who is about 67 years old just had one herself. She is a very avid smoker. She has some stents put into her arm but she refuses to give up smoking even though it is a detriment to her health. She has a large family of about 4 adult children and several grandkids who visit her. She is divorced and has a full life. Still, she is not willing to give up the awful habit of smoking. Her voice also sounds like a person who has been smoking for years sounding very husky. She also has a persistent cough, but will not give up smoking, even though it is the major cause of her medical condition. She had to be rushed to the hospital once in an ambulance due to her having a heart attack. Following that episode, I saw her in our building lobby and she seemed very frail. Still, her addiction to cigarettes she is willing to live with. In her mind, the pleasure and addition of smoking outweigh her having a good quality of life.

Another friend had a father-in-law who jogged every single day. He was retired and elderly still he kept up his great routine of jogging every day. One day he did not return from his run and was found lying lifeless on the road. He had succumbed to a heart attack. He was healthy as a horse.

To take care of your health, and to try to prevent a heart attack, stay away from fatty foods, avoid fried foods, don't consume a lot of junk food, exercise daily, and if you smoke, please get rid of that habit as it can cause a heart attack and/or a stroke which can be fatal. And that's the last thing you need in your busy and productive life. You want to enjoy your time on this earth. The more a person lives a healthy lifestyle, the more apt they are to continue to have a good quality of life, the less medical problems they will have, and, subsequently, make less trips to their family physician or the emergency room at their nearby hospital.

Chapter 18
Loneliness

In 2019 there are more and more people who live alone. There are a lot of children being raised by single mothers. A lot of millennials are also living alone. Most people tend to stay in contact via social media, texting, or email. There is not a lot of face to face interaction. If you look down your bus or your subway train when commuting to and from work or school you will see most people engrossed in their cellphones. Most will have their heads bent over and their backs hunched which poses another problem. With this constant bending over they are causing **kyphosis** which is the technical term for a hunch back. In recent weeks, it has been disclosed by the media that young people are growing bone spurs in the back of their heads, due to the incessant bending of the head they are doing while using cellphones.

The problem of loneliness has been seeping into Western society in recent years. Most people are having less contact with their friends, peers, or family. They may be at home watching Netflix or using Tinder for quick meet ups to have sex but not have a relationship with substance.

Loneliness is one of the worst things we can feel as humans. As babies, we need that human touch from our parents, especially our mothers, to survive. It has been found that babies who lack this connection from their mothers do not survive for very long.

A lot of elderly people don't have a lot of friends or family. Either their friends or family have died, or the ones they do have, do not stay in contact. On social media like Facebook we see a lot of curated lives of happiness but that is not really the case. (I've noticed there is a certain amount of people on Twitter, who post things almost daily, which sounds like they are depressed, and are unhappy in their relationships, and with life in general.) I've had some friends who have told me, that all that happiness I see in their pictures on Facebook, is not really the case in real life. Their spouse may get on their case or their parents or siblings treat them awfully. Their children may also not seem as happy-go-lucky as they appear in all those pictures. I have also a very large percentage of my Facebook friends in their 20s, 30s, 40s, 50s, and 60s, who do not have a significant other. Most of them are usually by themselves and almost all of them live alone. This follows the norm of what is happening in our society.

And loneliness is a silent killer. We need that human connection to maintain our happiness and well-being. You can still be in a room full of people and still feel very lonely. Humans are social beings and we need to have relations with other humans. The seniors who have happy lives usually have social interactions with people like going out of coffee, playing tennis, playing bridge or euchre, having chess clubs, going travelling with a friend or family member, going to the parties held by their friends or family. I have an elderly friend named Stan. He is retired but still drives a school bus. He actually took a European trip this year. He also had a summer party because he told me, "I would like to see my friends one last time before they put me in the ground." I attended his party but couldn't stay very long as I had a family emergency and sung karaoke with him. I could see he was having a blast. It was a very enjoyable party and I could see that Stan was having the time of his life. He has also taken tap dancing and is now taking piano lessons in his golden years. He also goes to the gym regularly. (Sorry, I know I'm repeating this bit from a previous chapter but I just want to emphasize how good it is to stay active and to socialize.) I really admire him for wanting to stay active during his twilight years.

We might think that because someone is rich and famous, they may not be lonely. Not true. Some of them because of their wealth and fame attract a lot of false friends who are only after their money or prestige. Some very wealthy people are terribly lonely. Her Royal Highness Princess Wilhelmina of the Netherlands once wrote a book entitled *Lonely but Not Alone* which was published in 1959, and goes to show that you can be surrounded by a lot of people, but still feel the awful chasm of loneliness.

If you presently live alone, try to join a book club, or make a concerted effort to socialize with some close friends or family. If you're able-bodied join some group of interest like a movie group, a gardening club, take trips with groups where you can forge some friendships, join a tennis club, or just go for a walk with a neighbor with whom you get along. Or start an investment or lottery group. That is a form of socializing. There were some seniors who started an investment group and they became so skilled that they started to make some money. Or maybe start an amateur theater group whereby you can then take your production to your city's fringe festival, and make some money, which can help with some of your household expenses. Or join a comedy club in your city. Some productions tend to see the light of day. I know Second City does this in some big cities. Or try your hand at stand-up comedy if you're very brave. I also know some elderly people who take regular bus trips to casinos which includes lunch. They don't gamble a lot but like the outing and to socialize with their fellow passengers.

Socializing requires some skill. A person must learn to listen as well as when to talk. If a person talks too much without listening to the other person, they are more apt to annoy the person they are with. Ask questions, inquire about the other person's life. **I would say speak 40% of the time and listen 60% of the time.** If you have one person who just talks and talks incessantly without trying to listen to the other person that will pose a problem. I've seen that being the case with some colleagues and their friends. It is very disconcerting when one person just wants to talk on and on without even inquiring about another person's life. Everyone likes to listen and also to be heard. It's human nature. That is also the basis about we learn things in life.

Whatever you do, quit segregating yourself from other people. Have an active social life and get out and meet people and experience the world. It will do much to boost your mental well-being, please your soul, and boost your confidence. You will then start to feel part of humanity not just someone who goes to work every day and comes home to an empty house or apartment. If you live like a hermit that will have a negative effect on your health and mental well-being.

Chapter 19
Calamine Lotion

Calamine lotion is one of the most under-rated products on the market. It can save you a trip to the emergency room or your local medical clinic. It's a pink liquid which you can purchase as an over the counter product at your local pharmacy.

It's great for a lot of skin rashes like bee stings, insect bites, heat rashes, poison ivy, measles, mosquito bites, or sun burns. It's quick and easy to use. You can use it on your pets, children, or your spouse. Just be sure if you place it on your pet they can't lick if off as it could be toxic. That being said, my wife and I have used it on our cat, whenever he gets seasonal allergies on his face (rashes which itch him like crazy), which the vet can't seem to help with. It works wonders on the little guy.

When a rash appears on your arms, face, legs, or body, you simply apply the calamine lotion and in one day's time it will alleviate any itchiness, discoloration, or small red bumps from rashes. The lotion is pink and has a powdery appearance. You can leave it on while you sleep. It will dissipate by morning and you can wash off the excess in the shower.

I just had a heat rash the other day on my fore arm and from my elbows down to my wrist my entire arm was covered in tiny little red bumps. My wife applied it to my fore arm just before bed and by the morning all the tiny little red bumps had become history. That took only one evening. She applied it around 8pm and by 6:30am when I awoke, all the red bumps on my arms had disappeared.

Calamine is not expensive and you can even buy the generic brand of the lotion. It even works on rashes or insect bites your cat or dogs may get, from being out on your balcony, or outside exploring your backyard or the neighborhood.

I never used it until I got married to my wife. She swears by it and it works like magic. Every medicine cabinet in every home should have a bottle of calamine lotion. It's one of those magic products most doctors or pharmacists don't tell you about.

Chapter 20
Medicinal Cannabis

There are several states in the United States which have legalized cannabis for medicinal as well as recreational use. Their neighbor to the north, Canada, has also legalized it across the board for both recreational use and for medicinal use. When a person suffers from such medical conditions as PTSD (post-traumatic-stress-disorder), multiple sclerosis (MS), anxiety, sleeping disorders, fibromyalgia, or any number of other issues, sometimes cannabis can be of help if modern medicine and other treatments are not helping the patient. CDB (cannabidiol) is not the active ingredient which makes a person high but can produce relief for some sufferers of some ailments.

The active ingredient THC (Tetrahydrocannabinol) is what makes people high when they smoke cannabis. It too does provide some relief for some suffers of some ailments, and can help to induce sleep in some suffers of a variety of illnesses, which modern medicine can't help. There are edible forms of cannabis containing THC or CDB if a person chooses not to smoke it. These edible forms should be kept out of reach of children and stored away properly. A child ingesting edible cannabis can get really sick and might have to be rushed to the emergency room.

I am all for whatever helps people who suffer from any ailments because suffering is not beneficial for having a good quality of life. And everyone deserves that.

THC in cannabis also has its drawback. It does slow down a person's reaction time and long-term use can lead to memory loss in some people. Some emergency room doctors have – since the legalization of cannabis – according to media reports have been suffering from psychosis after smoking cannabis. That being said, a person should not operate dangerous equipment like chainsaws, use knives, conveyor belts, barbeques, or drive after smoking cannabis with THC. It could lead to accidents which may be fatal.

In Colorado, the number of vehicular accidents has also increased since the legalization of cannabis. In addition, in Colorado, there have been some people who have experienced spontaneous vomiting which doctors could not explain until they traced back this phenomenon to the introduction of cannabis into every day usage.

If cannabis does help a person's ailment, I'm all for it. But, for younger people under the age of 25 when the human brain has not fully developed, they should not smoke cannabis. This can alter their brain chemistry leading to things like psychosis and even schizophrenia. I once saw a gentleman on a TV news program, who now is now a counsellor and advocate against cannabis use. He was initially for it but the young people he sees, most of them have developed psychosis, due to excessive cannabis use.

If you wish to consume cannabis, please do so under a doctor's supervision. So, he or she can gauge how it may change your personality or mental condition via close monitoring. It may not adversely affect it but then again it can. The THC in cannabis can and does affect each individual differently.

I also had friends I went to high school with who used cannabis. One smoked it into his late teens and well into his twenties, he smoked cannabis every day. By the time her had turned 30, his memory was impaired. He could not recall a lot of the many fun things we did as teenagers. They were all completely wiped from his memory. I had another high school friend who smoked cannabis to dull his senses. He could not cope with the adult world and lost his drive and his direction in life. All his friends were studying in college or university and getting on with their lives. He however had chosen to drop out of university. He eventually committed suicide by jumping off a bridge. He was very tall and good-looking and chose to end his life tragically. His death affected his parents and his only sibling greatly as they had many hopes and dreams for him. Another friend, used cannabis sparingly, but ended up having psychosis which was later cured after several years of counseling, pills, and therapy.

If you choose to use cannabis recreationally, be certain you know what you're doing. If you see changes in your health both physically or mentally, it might be time you stop using it. And remember if you're ingesting anything into your lungs, it could later lead to cancer. Your lungs were not meant to ingest smoke, only the air we breath. Take it from a person who has seen what it did to some of his friends.

Chapter 21
Counseling -- Grief or Alcohol

When we lose someone, we love in our lives, that is one of the most trying times in our lives. The loss will be almost unbearable to some. I had a friend whose 20-something year old son died unexpectedly. He was a very good-looking young man, with a lot of friends, and a lot of promise in life. He wanted to become a police officer to help people. His death has left my friend inconsolable for over four years now. She cries every day hoping that her son did not die and would somehow come back. We all know that is not going to happen. But there is nothing she can do to change that fact. I've talked her through it too many times, but she has cut me off entirely from her life choosing not to return my emails, and has decided to deal with it on her own. She is divorced and has no support network. Her relationship with her siblings is strained at best. All she does is lock herself in her home, watch movies, and cries almost non-stop. She will no longer return my calls. Once I had to send police officers to check on her in the middle of the night because she would not respond to my calls. Fortunately, she was alright. I am truly her only friend. All of her other friends have abandoned her. I am the only one who remembers her birthday and sends her well wishes. No one else does.

I have encouraged her to see a psychologist or psychiatrist or join a grief counseling group. She was involved in a counseling group at one point but did not find it beneficial. She wants to deal with her immense loss all on her own. That crux of the matter is, if someone does not wish to seek help, help may not be forthcoming. There is an adage that goes: you can't help someone who does not want to be helped.

I encourage you if you are grieving the loss of a loved one and do not have good support network of friends and family, to please seek a bereavement group. It will help you. When we deal with others who can relate to our suffering it does help. Others who are suffering from the same problems, can understand better, and empathize more than people who are not in the same boat.

Same goes for people who are suffering from alcoholism. Some of us tend to start consuming beer, wine or spirits to try to numb us from the issues we have to deal with every day and the stresses of every day life. Issues such as a divorce, friction with our siblings, loss of a job, issues with our coworkers, a difficult boss, and maybe money problems. That comes as a part of being human and trying to live in a very complex society. That all plays on our mental health. If you, or someone you know, is suffering from alcoholism which can lead to cirrhosis of the liver, which could make your problems even worst, I would implore you or your friend or relative to seek alcohol counseling. The best as we know is Alcoholics Anonymous. They have done wonders for helping people who only find solace in the bottle. They have helped millions and can help you overcome the issues you deal with every day.

Some people who drink to drown their sorrows, may even go into work inebriated, which could lead to the loss of their jobs, which could only make their situation even worst.

I would behoove you whether it's grief you're suffering from or an addiction to alcohol, please seek help, because it will make a world of difference. You may not see it now that you're mired in your problem, but when you start meeting others who suffer from the same condition, it will make a huge difference in your life. Get help. I wish you all the best in your recovery.

Take it from someone who use to drink to excess. I did it in my early twenties. Then one day I just quit cold turkey. I asked myself, "What are you really doing? Does drinking to excess really make you happy? What are you accomplishing but making a fool of yourself?" That did it. I am more of a social drinker now. At home I might have a glass of wine with dinner occasionally and have maybe 4 beers over the course of a year. I get much more pleasure from drinking coffee or tea now. Those are my only vice.

Concerning the grief part, I have lost several friends and older relatives within the last 4 or 5 years. I also lost a pet which was an integral part of my family. I did not go for counseling but I had a good network of family and friends who provided it for me. Talking about it with loved ones is just like counseling. Talk therapy either with a professional or family or friends is cathartic.

Chapter 22
Weight Loss

There are really two magic bullets when it comes to weight loss. Most people don't consider them but they are the only two logical solutions. Yes, there is Weight Watchers, the Atkins Diet, the Keto Diet, and Jenny Craig, plus numerous other weight loss programs that come and go. Most which can be very expensive. However, with a good concerted effort many people would be saving a lot of money if they only act logically.

First, you have to get exercise. A lot of people with weight issues don't exercise very much but consume a lot of calories. That is their first big problem. Plus, they may snack during the day while also having breakfast, lunch, and dinner. I knew two young ladies who had amazing figures but gained a lot of weight as they approach their thirties because they just ate too much. They had food at their desks and ate all day while working. Also, you've probably heard about the "freshman 15"? That is, freshmen in university or college usually gain 15 lbs. during their first year of college or university. I've seen it happen numerous times. What can that be attributed to? Eating too much and not getting enough exercise. Add drinking beer or alcohol to the mix and that's a lot of calories each student is adding to their diet each day.

So, people consuming too much calories during the day and eating way too much and possibly junk food as well adds extra pounds. And if they drive to and from work that's another way to put on the extra pounds.

Next, portion control when a person eats. Don't go for the buffet if you go to a restaurant and eat like you're at a trough. If you do opt for the buffet, have a little of each entrée. Don't eat as much as you can until you get bloated. That's a huge problem in most restaurant: they give a patron too much food to dine on. I ate at a number of restaurants while in the United

States on three different trips and I was astounded how much food they give. The appetizers were large enough for a meal.

The crown and glory are to get exercise. Whether by walking, using weights, or joining a gym. Most people are too lackadaisical about exercise but still enjoy eating a lot. If you love food you've got to shed those pounds.

There are a few people who live in my condo building. Both men and women. There are about 10 all in excess of 200 lbs. The problem with them is they get zero exercise each day. They drive to and from work, they drive to the grocery store, they drive to the corner store, they drive to the movies, they drive to restaurants, they drive to visit family, they even drive to the local coffee shop which is a block away, and don't get any exercise. And I've known most of these people for ten years! All that time they have gotten no exercise. And we have a free gym in our building!!! The only time they got exercise was when our elevators were out of service and they had to walk up and down the stairs. The issue is they've been that way most of their lives, so they don't see any need to change and, most importantly, lack the drive.

I also know about several people who are over 200 lbs. who I associate with. There are about 8 of them. Some are close to 200 or 300 lbs. Over a 10-year period only one had has shed about 80 lbs. Her name is Philippa. How did she do it? She controlled the portions that she eats and most of all she has taken up exercising.

I also knew Amy during high school. She was close to 200 lbs. throughout high school. Now, she's middle-age and she is about 120 lbs. How did she do it? She exercises and run marathons. I've got to admit both Amy and Philippa look great and I am so happy for them.

I also knew Serge during junior high and high school. He used to weight about 350 lbs. He is about 180 lbs. now. He also too has taken up an exercise regimen which has served him well. He does a lot of cycling. I was so glad to see him years after high school and how he had transformed his physique.

So, you don't have to pay for an expensive weight loss program. All you have to do is keep your portions at each meal very small within reason (so you don't starve), watch the calories you eat, and, most of all, get exercise every single day. I, too, had put on some extra pounds when I started working after college, which I shed because I was eating more, and stopped playing sports. I had to change that habit and fast! Good luck to you!

Chapter 23
Age Spots

As we age some of us will start to get dark spots on our face or a slight discoloration. Those are commonly referred to as age spots. They might be slightly dark in color which will be or might be circular or oval in nature. Some of those age spots might be lighter in color but take over a larger portion of your face. This affects anyone regardless of ethnicity whether you're Caucasian, Asian, South Asian, or of African descent.

Nivea is a cream which will help. It might not totally take away the age spots but will lessen their darkness. Nivea is made by a German company which also produces another cream which lightens your skin, said to be a huge seller in countries like India.

So, if you're getting age spots, no matter how young or old you are, buy some Nivea, and apply it to your face before you sleep at night. Rub it in so it does not leave marks on your pillow. It will lessen the darkness of your age spots. But you must do it every night.

I started to get some discoloration on my face when I reached my late thirties. Something viscerally gravitated me to Nivea. I then learned in an article in the New York Times, that Nivea is made by the same aforesaid company which makes skin lightening cream.

Nivea is not all that expensive and can be bought over the counter. I would suggest you buy some if you're starting to get age spots on your face. The other option may be laser surgery but that is more expensive. Take care of your skin and it will take care of you because you want to look beautiful for as long as you can.

Final Words

Some last suggestions. Eat blueberries to benefit your eyes. Most of us start to need glasses either for reading or distances when we turn 40. Blueberries may delay that.

Walnuts are good for your brain, so grab a handful every day. In fact, all nuts are good also for their fiber for your health and to produce bowel movements. And having a handful of unsalted and not roasted almonds every day can keep your bad cholesterol at a good level. The dry kind are the best. When they are roasted their potency is diminished.

Spinach is a great source of calcium. So is milk and orange juice. But orange juice is high in sugar so consume it in moderation. Remember to also do the same for sodas. And if you're a vegan or vegetarian you still need your calcium. I would suggest you also research what other vegetables may be a good source of calcium, if you're vegan since you abstain from other dairy products, which are rich in calcium like yogurt and cheese.

Most of all get your requisite 7 or 8 hours of sleep every night, try to eat right, and get enough exercise every single day. And drink lots of water as our bodies are composed of mostly of water and we need water to benefit our overall makeup. Also, if you take medication or vitamins via a tablet, water by urinating will flush the excess from your system that your body does not use or need. And don't drink carbonated water, it is not as good as tap water or spring water from a bottle. I wish you well on maintaining good optimal health for your time on the earth.

Selected Sources:

1. "A Pain in the Head," an article by Women's College Hospital in the Toronto Star, Thursday, July 25, 2019, page T7.
2. Article: "The Science Behind Aging Well" from Toronto's Women's College Hospital in the Toronto Star, on page T7. Thursday, August 8, 2019. This article is sponsored content.
3. Article: "Fighting the plight of loneliness" by Dow Marmur (opinion piece). Monday, August 12, 2019. Toronto Star, page A11.
4. Op-ed: "Making a case for a national dental program" by Dr. Hazel Stewart. Toronto Star, pg. A11. Monday, August 19, 2019.

About the author: Michael Persaud is a freelance writer, poet, and author. He likes to take an active role in taking care of his health. He has read voluminous amounts of articles on medical innovations and treatments over the last 32 years. During that time, he has also seen numerous medical reports and news programs on what is happening in the world of medicine. He served two terms as the president of The Ontario Poetry Society (TOPS). He has also worked in the field of tourism for over two decades and is a certified travel agent. He would like to extend his gratitude to you for purchasing this book. He was a former music critic and reviewer for his college newspaper. He has worked for a mystery shopping company and also for a company which ran medical clinics. He also worked as a restaurant reviewer for a community newspaper. He has written for numerous publications including the largest newspaper in Canada, by circulation, the Toronto Star, The Downsview Advocate, Equality, Afterword, Write Magazine (now defunct – this publication was not affiliated with the Writers' Union of Canada), Eye Weekly (now defunct), and The Outreach Connection. He loves trivia and loves to watch Jeopardy when time permits. If you liked this book you might also like to try one of his other titles:

The Ultimate Trivia Book

Random Facts About Rock Music's Greatest Acts

… continued

True Paranormal Stories: Stories You Will Have to Read in Order to Believe

Ottawa Travel Guide

Calgary Travel Guide

Winnipeg Travel Guide

90 Awesome Things to do in Toronto!

How to Win the Lottery!: Playing to Win and Winning More Often!

1,004 Random Facts and Amazing Trivia: Impress Your Family & Friends with What You Know!

800 Ultimate Trivia Questions

Ultimate Rock and Roll Trivia

How to Improve Your Vocabulary, Writing, and English in Less Than 30 Days

How to Write Faster When You Have a Full-time Job

Massive Movie Trivia

Toronto: A Complete Guide on the City

Totally Random Movie Trivia

The Beatles

The Amazing Trivia Book

Great Names in the World of Popular Music: From the 50's to the 90's

Inspirational Quotes for Every Day of the Year

Viva Morrissey

Adele: Voice of an Angel

Essential New York: A Tourist Guide on the City

How to Make Even More Money: Learning the Tricks That Will Get You Ahead

A Montreal Travel Guide

How to Find a Job in Hard Times

How to Win Friends Easily

How to Save More Money

A Canadian Childhood

Made in United States
Orlando, FL
08 December 2023

40460251R00093